T0302901

# Readiness of Soldiers and Adult Family Members Who Receive Behavioral Health Care

Identifying Promising Outcome Metrics

KIMBERLY A. HEPNER, CAROL P. ROTH, HEATHER KRULL, LEA XENAKIS, HAROLD ALAN PINCUS

Prepared for the United States Army
Approved for public release; distribution unlimited

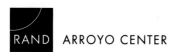

For more information on this publication, visit **www.rand.org/t/RR4268**.

**About RAND**

The RAND Corporation is a research organization that develops solutions to public policy challenges to help make communities throughout the world safer and more secure, healthier and more prosperous. RAND is nonprofit, nonpartisan, and committed to the public interest. To learn more about RAND, visit www.rand.org.

**Research Integrity**

Our mission to help improve policy and decisionmaking through research and analysis is enabled through our core values of quality and objectivity and our unwavering commitment to the highest level of integrity and ethical behavior. To help ensure our research and analysis are rigorous, objective, and nonpartisan, we subject our research publications to a robust and exacting quality-assurance process; avoid both the appearance and reality of financial and other conflicts of interest through staff training, project screening, and a policy of mandatory disclosure; and pursue transparency in our research engagements through our commitment to the open publication of our research findings and recommendations, disclosure of the source of funding of published research, and policies to ensure intellectual independence. For more information, visit www.rand.org/about/principles.

RAND's publications do not necessarily reflect the opinions of its research clients and sponsors.

Published by the RAND Corporation, Santa Monica, Calif.
© 2021 RAND Corporation
RAND® is a registered trademark.

Library of Congress Cataloging-in-Publication Data is available for this publication.
ISBN: 978-1-9774-0480-0

# Preface

This report documents research and analysis conducted as part of the project entitled *Ready Soldiers and Families: Identifying Metrics of Readiness Following Behavioral Health Care*, sponsored by the Office of the Surgeon General, U.S. Army Medical Command. The purpose of the project was to identify metrics to assess soldier and family readiness following behavioral health care to support the Army's efforts to monitor and improve behavioral health care.

This research was conducted within RAND Arroyo Center's Personnel, Training, and Health Program. RAND Arroyo Center, part of the RAND Corporation, is a federally funded research and development center (FFRDC) sponsored by the United States Army.

RAND operates under a "Federal-Wide Assurance" (FWA00003425) and complies with the *Code of Federal Regulations for the Protection of Human Subjects Under United States Law* (45 CFR 46), also known as "the Common Rule," as well as with the implementation guidance set forth in DoD Instruction 3216.02. As applicable, this compliance includes reviews and approvals by RAND's Institutional Review Board (the Human Subjects Protection Committee) and by the U.S. Army. The views of sources utilized in this study are solely their own and do not represent the official policy or position of DoD or the U.S. government.

# Contents

# Figures and Boxes

# Tables

# Summary

*The research reported here was completed in February 2020, followed by security review by the sponsor and the Office of the Chief of Public Affairs, with final sign-off in August 2021.*

Behavioral health (BH) conditions, such as posttraumatic stress disorder (PTSD), depression, and anxiety, are the second most common medical reason for nondeployability in the U.S. Army. Force readiness is tied not only to individual soldiers' health but also to the well-being of their families. For these reasons, the health and readiness of soldiers and their families is a top concern for the Army, as is ensuring that soldiers and their families have access to high-quality, effective BH care.

A chief strategy that the Army uses to monitor and improve BH treatment is to assess changes in psychological symptoms experienced over the course of BH specialty care. It does so by tracking the proportion of patients who have experienced clinically significant decreases in symptoms. Although such symptom-based metrics are useful, metrics that specifically assess soldier and family readiness could further strengthen the Army's awareness of soldiers' BH treatment outcomes and their readiness to deploy.

To support its efforts to monitor and improve BH care, the Army asked RAND Arroyo Center, part of the RAND Corporation, to identify promising metrics to assess readiness among soldiers and adult family members who receive BH care. Ideally, such metrics would capture whether soldiers and their adult family members returned to a high level of functioning following treatment. Thus, the goal of these metrics would be to expand the Army's outcome monitoring efforts beyond symptoms to include one or more readiness-related metrics, providing additional information to assess and improve the effectiveness of BH care.

Although this project was conducted for the Army, the findings and recommendations will likely be of interest to a broader audience across service branches and the military medical community.

## Assessing the Behavioral Health Needs of Soldiers and Their Families and Identifying Metrics to Monitor Readiness

BH diagnoses are common across the U.S. military. Among all active-duty service members, 20 percent received a BH diagnosis through the Military Health System (MHS) in fiscal year (FY) 2016, with the highest within-service-branch proportion being in the Army (26 percent compared with 15–18 percent for other service branches). This pattern was similar for rates of anxiety, depression, and PTSD diagnoses (Deployment Health Clinical Center, 2017).

Deployments and postdeployment reintegration can be stressful for both service members and their families. A recent survey of 9,845 married couples across service branches found that 36 percent of spouses met criteria for at least one psychiatric condition (Steenkamp et al., 2018). In a convenience sample of 171 Army and Marine Corps families, 15–25 percent of spouses experienced symptoms of stress, anxiety, and depression during their service member's deployment; 10–18 percent of spouses whose service member had recently returned from a deployment experienced these symptoms (Lester et al., 2010). Although spouses were more willing to seek help for their BH problems than soldiers, their main source of BH care was their on-post primary care clinic rather than a BH specialty care provider (Eaton et al., 2008).

A core component of soldier readiness is the ability to deploy. Soldiers who have a temporary or permanent medical condition that may render them not medically ready to deploy are put on a *profile*. In 2017, the Army issued a memorandum to standardize the application of profiles for BH conditions to appropriately inform commanders of duty limitations and treatment support recommendations. The memorandum instructs health care providers to assess soldiers' medical readiness for duty during every clinical encounter.

There are a variety of definitions of soldier and family readiness. For the purpose of this project, we defined these concepts as follows:

- soldier readiness: the ability to perform mission-essential tasks and deploy without limitations from a BH condition
- family readiness: the state of being prepared to effectively navigate the challenges of daily living experienced in the unique context of military service, to include mobility and financial readiness, mobilization and deployment readiness, and personal and family life readiness.

Although the U.S. Department of Defense (DoD) definition of family readiness could apply to children, adolescents, and the family as a whole, this report considered only adult family members who receive BH care. The Army aims to provide timely access to high-quality BH care for both soldiers and their families. Monitoring symptom improvement provides valuable information about the effectiveness of Army BH care and the proportion of patients whose symptoms improve. Yet existing metrics do not fully capture whether soldiers and adult family members achieve readiness after receiving BH care. Incorporating one or more readiness metrics into its outcome monitoring process would provide a clearer picture of readiness levels for those who receive Army BH care.

It is important to select metrics that are reliable, directly relevant to the domain of care that is being measured, and sensitive to changes in care. Choosing the wrong metrics could lead to costly implementation and results that are not useful. However, even when an appropriate outcome metric has been selected, implementation could be associated with an increased burden for staff who must administer and incorporate the metric into the care provided and for patients who may need to spend time completing self-report measures. For these reasons, metrics that are intended to drive quality improvement have associated costs that need to be balanced with the potential gains.

## Project Methods

We developed a set of criteria to use as a basis for evaluating candidate readiness metrics. These criteria were adapted from those used by the National Quality Forum to evaluate quality measures submitted for its potential endorsement (National Quality Forum, 2018). Characteristics of a desirable readiness metric include the following:

- *Importance.* Does the metric address a high-priority area in which performance could improve?
- *Feasibility.* Do the data exist to measure metric performance? Are those data accessible without undue burden?
- *Scientific acceptability.* Is the metric reliable and valid in measuring the area of interest? Is it sensitive to change?
- *Usability.* Do providers view the metric as useful and informative in assessing BH care?

To inform our assessment, we conducted interviews with stakeholders, reviewed the range of existing sources of data that could support the development of a readiness metric, and conducted an instrument search to identify and evaluate instruments that have been used to measure readiness-related domains in both military and civilian populations.

### Stakeholder Interviews

To obtain stakeholder perspectives on soldier and family readiness, we conducted interviews with Army BH subject-matter experts and Army BH providers. We solicited the perspectives of these experts and providers on conceptual indicators of readiness. These perspectives provided important information about which aspects of readiness should be captured in a readiness metric. We also gained insight into how BH providers currently assess readiness and solicited suggestions from both BH experts and providers on how readiness assessment could be improved.

Eligible Army BH experts included Army personnel who had participated in designing policies around readiness, assessed BH care quality or outcomes, been involved in designing systems that capture information to assess soldier or family readiness, or participated in BH quality monitoring and improvement activities. Army

BH providers were eligible to participate if they delivered BH treatment to soldiers or family members at an Army military treatment facility (MTF). Providers could have worked in a variety of BH settings, such as Embedded Behavioral Health and BH specialty clinics. Eligible provider types included psychiatrists, psychologists, master's-level clinicians, and counselors. In total, we interviewed 18 BH experts and 24 BH providers. For both groups, participation was optional. The Army provided a list of potential BH experts, and installation directors of BH were tasked with identifying potential BH provider participants.

### Review of Existing Data Sources

We reviewed existing data sources to determine whether data elements that are currently collected and housed in military systems could support a soldier or family member readiness metric. We considered the content of each data source and its direct applicability to measuring readiness. For each data source, we considered the appropriateness of the variables for potential use in a readiness metric.

The Army currently monitors the BH care provided to soldiers in MTFs using data from the Behavioral Health Data Portal (BHDP). Most BHDP instruments assess symptomology that may affect readiness and inform treatment, but they do not address the broader construct of readiness. However, we identified the Walter Reed Functional Impairment Scale (WRFIS) as a promising instrument to use as the basis for developing a soldier readiness metric. The WRFIS was also suggested by two of the BH experts we interviewed.

A key benefit of the instrument is that it was developed specifically for use with active-duty military personnel, a population that faces unique occupational physical demands and opportunities for exposure to stressful events (see Herrell et al., 2014). Table S.1 shows a step-by-step approach to pilot testing a WRFIS-based readiness metric.

**Table S.1**
**Plan for Pilot Testing a WRFIS-Based Readiness Metric**

| Step | Description | Goal |
|------|-------------|------|
| 1 | Assess current extent to which the WRFIS is used for Army BH care | Determine the level of effort that will be needed to reach full implementation |
| 2 | Conduct descriptive analyses of existing WRFIS data | Evaluate psychometric properties of the WRFIS among soldiers who receive BH care and inform outcome metric specifications |
| 3 | Define detailed metric specifications | Develop detailed outcome metric specifications to increase the likelihood that the metric meets evaluation criteria (e.g., scientific acceptability) |
| 4 | Pilot test metric | Assess whether the metric provides useful data on readiness and can be used to monitor and improve BH care |

A second potential source on which to base a readiness metric is eProfile, the data system that the Army uses to track soldiers who have a temporary or permanent medical condition that may make them medically unready for a deployment. There are policies and guidance on when and how to assign a soldier a temporary or permanent profile, including the recently implemented Behavioral Health Readiness Evaluation and Decisionmaking Instrument (B-REDI), a decision support tool designed to help providers determine whether to write a profile for a soldier for a BH condition. Nonetheless, our interview respondents reported a lack of consistency in how profiles are applied, something that could limit the utility of profile data as a source for a readiness metric. Potential inconsistency also points to a need for continued training and decision support for providers on when and how to place a soldier on a profile.

### Instrument Search

We conducted a search of the peer-reviewed literature to identify instruments that have been used to assess the readiness of soldiers or adult family members. There are many components that affect readiness (e.g., social support, financial constraints, family issues, mental and physical health), so we aimed to identify a single instrument that would support a readiness metric capable of assessing multiple components of readiness. Our search focused on instruments that could capture the unique demands on soldiers and their families.

To remain in consideration, an instrument needed to assess readiness, be self-report, and contain no more than 30 items. Few instruments met all of these standards. We identified two potentially promising instruments that measured resilience, but both instruments were proprietary tools. Ultimately, we found that none of the instruments in the literature that had been used with military populations or their families met our final inclusion criteria for further consideration.

We also conducted a supplemental search for recommended instruments that measure functioning—a concept related to readiness—in the civilian population. Despite identifying three potentially useful instruments that assess health status and disability in both clinical and population settings, we determined that they were not as relevant to soldiers and their families, who are younger, on average, than the civilian population and face unique stressors. Therefore, none of the instruments identified in our supplemental search met final inclusion criteria for further consideration.

## Findings

There are several strengths associated with the methods we employed, but our project also had some limitations. First, we focused only on the readiness of soldiers and adult family members. The readiness of children and adolescents and the family as a unit is also a key part of overall family readiness. Second, policies related to readiness vary across service branches. Our project was limited to Army policies, personnel, and families, and our interviews were limited to Army BH experts and providers. Therefore, our findings may not be applicable to other service branches. Third, we conducted a limited number of interviews, and few respondents had experience working with adult family members. Fourth, we were unable to include planned interviews with commanders, and therefore that perspective is lacking. Further, the perspectives of soldiers and adult family members were not included. Finally, because readiness represents a unique type of functioning in the military community, we applied strictly defined criteria to guide our instrument search. Therefore, we may have missed some sources that may have warranted consideration.

### Stakeholders Reported That Psychiatric Symptoms, Diagnoses, Treatment, and Impaired Functioning Are Important Indicators of Lack of Readiness for Soldiers and Adult Family Members

When asked about conceptual indicators of readiness, BH experts and BH providers cited psychiatric symptoms or diagnoses and related treatment as indicators of not being ready for both soldiers and adult family members. These included psychiatric symptoms related to risk (e.g., suicidal ideation) and specific BH diagnoses (e.g., PTSD, depression, substance use disorder) with high symptom severity, need for intensive psychiatric treatment, or treatment with certain psychotropic medications. These responses reflected the Army's current policies regarding BH conditions and their potential negative impact on readiness. Findings from our stakeholder interviews highlighted the importance of ongoing symptom monitoring as a key component of monitoring readiness for soldiers and adult family members.

Input regarding conceptual indicators of readiness also highlighted the important role of multiple aspects of functioning, including occupational functioning (particularly for soldiers), social functioning, and general functioning (particularly for family members) related to readiness. Although there are numerous instruments that assess functioning in general populations, in the case of the Army, the challenge of identifying a metric of functioning is complicated by the unique demands the military places on soldiers and their adult family members.

### No Existing Data Source or Patient Self-Report Instrument Met Criteria for Army-Wide Implementation of a Readiness Metric for Soldiers, but One Instrument Is Promising

We used rigorous criteria to evaluate whether any existing data sources would support a readiness metric for soldiers and/or adult family members. The WRFIS assesses important components of soldier readiness, is feasible to use, and appears valid and reliable (based on the psychometric properties of the original form). Unfortunately, there are no data about its sensitivity to change (i.e., whether scores improve over time in response to effective treatment) or its usability as a clinical tool for providers to inform care for individual patients. Therefore, some additional work is needed before it could be implemented on a large scale. Once these parameters are established, a pilot would be a useful way to test whether the WRFIS could support a soldier readiness metric.

### No Existing Data Source or Patient Self-Report Instrument Met Criteria for Army-Wide Implementation of a Readiness Metric for Adult Family Members

Neither the WRFIS nor any other data source or instrument we evaluated would support a readiness metric for adult family members. The demands of military readiness on families are unique compared with the functional demands of civilian populations. Instruments to measure functioning in general populations tend to focus on self-care and activity limitations related to physical and mental health problems, making them less relevant to military adult family members who are likely to be young and in generally good health. In addition, the development of instruments to measure overall functioning, including in the context of BH care, is still evolving. Therefore, we found no existing self-report instrument to recommend for Army-wide implementation to monitor family readiness at this time.

### BH Providers Reported Some Variability in Assessing Readiness, but BH Experts and Providers Offered Suggestions for Improving Readiness Assessment

BH providers reported using similar information to assess readiness, including occupational functioning, policy guidance, and such collateral information as consulting with the soldier's command and, to a lesser extent, friends and family. The most common information used to assess readiness, however, was patient self-report measures and clinical interviews, which providers use to assess the soldier's clinical presentation, determine diagnoses, and inform the treatment plan. Responses were more variable as to whether a soldier's specific duties informed the readiness decision and whether to place the soldier on a profile.

BH experts and BH providers had many suggestions for improving how readiness is assessed. Two specific ideas had the most support: BHDP should be improved and expanded to include additional measures and information about soldiers, and more information should be collected about family members.

## Recommendations and Policy Implications

### Recommendation 1. Conduct a Pilot Evaluation of a WRFIS-Based Soldier Readiness Metric

We found the WRFIS to be a viable option for further work to develop a soldier readiness metric. The WRFIS's specificity to soldier readiness and feasibility of use (brief length, currently available in BHDP, and accessible to providers and Defense Health Agency leadership) are notable strengths. Although the WRFIS is currently included in BHDP, we do not have current information about its level of use by providers or its clinical utility. We also did not identify an alternative instrument that was suitable for soldiers and had adequate psychometric properties. We recommend that the Army systematically test the use of the WRFIS. These analyses would guide the development of a potential metric to monitor soldier readiness that could be pilot tested in a defined population of those who receive Army BH care.

### Recommendation 2. Increase Standardization in Applying Profiles and Continue B-REDI Training

Profiles are used to communicate that a soldier has a medical condition that limits their ability to perform job-related duties. Therefore, we initially believed that profile data could potentially be used to develop a metric that assesses and tracks soldier readiness. However, we learned during interviews that there are issues with how BH profiles are applied. We recommend that, before the Army considers using profile data to develop a readiness metric, steps should be taken to ensure that profiles are applied consistently across providers. Providers should receive additional training on when and how to place a soldier on a profile and continue provider decision support efforts. The B-REDI tool and associated training are an excellent example of the Army's efforts to standardize the application of profiles, and this effort should be continued.

## Directions for Future Research

We identified several areas that could be addressed in future research, including the development of an instrument to assess readiness for adult family members. Another research direction would be to assess the utility of profile data, including the reliability and validity of these data and how the presence of a profile predicts soldier service and BH outcomes. In addition, it would be useful to identify an approach to assessing the readiness of service members across service branches who receive BH care from the MHS. Lastly, efforts should be made to capture stakeholder perspectives that were not represented in this report, specifically commanders and those who receive BH care.

# Acknowledgments

We gratefully acknowledge the support of our project sponsors, LTC Deborah Enger-ran, Kelly Woolaway-Bickel, and LTC Chester Jean in the Office of the Surgeon General, U.S. Army Medical Command. We appreciate the valuable insights we received from Carrie Farmer of RAND and Maria Steenkamp of New York University. We addressed their constructive critiques as part of RAND's rigorous quality assurance process to improve the quality of this report. We thank Lauren Skrabala for revisions to the report and Tiffany Hruby for report preparation. Finally, we are grateful to the Army BH subject-matter experts and providers who participated in this study, sharing both their time and experience.

# Abbreviations

| | |
|---|---|
| BH | behavioral health |
| BHDP | Behavioral Health Data Portal |
| B-REDI | Behavioral Health Readiness Evaluation and Decisionmaking Instrument |
| CAFBHS | Child and Family Behavioral Health Services |
| DHA | Defense Health Agency |
| DoD | U.S. Department of Defense |
| FORSCOM | U.S. Army Forces Command |
| FY | fiscal year |
| MBHR | Mental and Behavioral Health Registry |
| MDD | major depressive disorder |
| MEDCOM | U.S. Army Medical Command |
| MHS | Military Health System |
| MODS | Medical Operational Data System |
| MOS | military occupational specialty |
| MTF | military treatment facility |
| NQF | National Quality Forum |
| OTSG | Office of the Surgeon General |
| PHQ-9 | Patient Health Questionnaire |
| PROMIS | Patient-Reported Outcomes Measurement Information System |
| PTSD | posttraumatic stress disorder |
| PULHES | military medical grading system: P, physical capacity/stamina; U, upper extremities; L, lower extremities; H, hearing/ear; E, eyes; S, psychiatric |
| RADaR | Rapid and Rigorous Qualitative Data Analysis |
| SUD | substance use disorder |

| | |
|---|---|
| SUDCC | Substance Use Disorder Clinical Care |
| VR-12 | Veterans RAND 12-Item Health Survey |
| VTA | Veterans Tracking Application |
| WHODAS | World Health Organization Disability Assessment Schedule |
| WRFIS | Walter Reed Functional Impairment Scale |

# CHAPTER ONE

# Introduction

## Overview

The health and readiness of soldiers and their families is a top concern for the U.S. Army. Behavioral health (BH) conditions, such as posttraumatic stress disorder (PTSD) and depression, can potentially have a significant negative impact on readiness. Collectively, BH conditions are the second most common medical reason (after musculoskeletal problems) for not being ready to deploy (U.S. Army Public Health Center, 2018). Thus, access to high-quality, effective BH care is essential. One chief strategy that the Army uses to monitor and improve BH treatment is to assess changes in psychological symptoms experienced over the course of BH specialty care (Defense Health Agency, 2018). Specifically, the Army tracks the proportion of patients who experience clinically significant decreases in PTSD, depression, and anxiety symptoms. While these symptom-based metrics provide essential information about whether patients experience an improvement in symptoms associated with their diagnoses during BH treatment, metrics that specifically assess soldier and family readiness could strengthen the Army's monitoring of BH outcomes.

To support its readiness mission and its effort to monitor and improve BH care, the Army asked RAND Arroyo Center, part of the RAND Corporation, to identify metrics to assess readiness among soldiers and adult family members who receive BH care. Ideally, such metrics would capture whether soldiers and their adult family members return to a high level of functioning following treatment. Thus, the goal of these metrics would be to expand the Army's outcome monitoring efforts beyond symptoms to include one or more readiness-related metrics, providing additional information to assess and improve the effectiveness of BH care.

In this chapter, we first describe the Army's efforts to support soldier and family readiness in the context of BH care and then provide the definitions of readiness that were used for this project. Next, we provide an overview of quality measurement and improvement. Finally, we provide a description of the Army's current efforts to monitor and improve BH care and how a readiness-related outcome metric could strengthen these efforts.

Although this project was conducted for the Army, which guided its focus, the findings and recommendations in this report will be of broader interest to Defense Health Agency (DHA) leadership. The Military Health System (MHS) is in the process of consolidating the administration and management of all military treatment facilities under the DHA in a phased approach that is scheduled to be completed by October 2021 (Adirim, 2019). Because of these changes, the work presented here will be applicable to a broader audience across all service branches.

## Behavioral Health Needs of Soldiers and Their Families

Across service branches, there is a need for high-quality BH care for both service members and their families. Among all U.S. active-duty service members, 20 percent received a BH diagnosis through the MHS in FY 2016. When examined by service branch, data indicated that 26 percent of Army soldiers had a BH diagnosis compared with 15–18 percent of service members in other branches (Deployment Health Clinical Center, 2017). This pattern was echoed for rates of anxiety and depressive disorder diagnoses and PTSD diagnoses, which, at 7 percent and 4 percent, respectively, were higher in the Army than in the Air Force, Navy, or Marine Corps (Deployment Health Clinical Center, 2017). The U.S. Department of Defense (DoD) Health-Related Behaviors Survey collects self-report data from a sample of nondeployed active-component personnel. In 2015, almost 18 percent of respondents reported experiencing at least one of three mental health problems (probable depression, probable generalized anxiety disorder, and probable PTSD), and almost 10 percent reported experiencing two or more (Meadows et al., 2018). Deployments, which typically separate the soldier from his or her family, and eventual postdeployment reintegration can contribute further stressors.

Access to high-quality BH care is similarly critical for adult family members. Military spouses have shown higher levels of emotional distress across nine dimensions, including depression and anxiety, than their civilian counterparts (Lester et al., 2010). In a study of 940 soldiers' spouses who sought primary care or attended a family readiness group meeting, 20 percent met screening criteria for either major depression or anxiety disorder (Eaton et al., 2008). When a single-item functional impairment criterion was combined with diagnostic criteria, providing a more stringent threshold, rates of depression or generalized anxiety were 8 percent in this group. Spouses were more willing to seek help for their BH problems than soldiers, but their main source of BH care was their on-post primary care clinic (Eaton et al., 2008).

Deployments are a significant stressor for Army spouses. In a convenience sample of 171 Army and Marine Corps families, 15–25 percent of spouses experienced symptoms of stress, anxiety, and depression during their service member's deployment; 10–18 percent of spouses whose service member had recently returned from a deployment experienced these symptoms (Lester et al., 2010). In a more recent study, data from surveyed spouses of active-duty service members from all service branches, the National Guard, and the Reserve ($n = 9,845$) revealed that 36 percent met criteria for at least one psychiatric condition. Most commonly endorsed conditions were moderate to severe somatization symptoms (18 percent) and insomnia (16 percent) (Steenkamp et al., 2018). Poorer mental health of spouses of deployed service members is also significantly associated with a greater number of academic and psychosocial challenges for their children (Chandra et al., 2010).

## Rationale for Identifying Readiness-Related Outcome Metrics

### Defining Soldier and Family Readiness

There are a variety of definitions of soldier and family readiness; for this project, we adopted the definitions shown in Box 1.1. The Army has described the characteristics required for soldier readiness as including the capability to conduct all required military operations, as well as maintenance of multidomain fitness (e.g., physical, environmental, medical and dental, nutritional, spiritual, psychological, behavioral, and social) (Chairman of the Joint Chiefs of Staff Instruction 3405.01, 2011; Milley, 2016). Optimal functioning is important in the civilian population but, for soldiers, functional demands are higher and focus heavily on military occupational performance. In addition, soldier functional demands may vary over time, depending on the soldier's patterns of deployment. Army definitions also note that readiness extends beyond the soldier and includes strong family, community, and organizational resilience, highlighting the key role of family health (DoD Instruction 6025.19, 2014; Chairman of the Joint Chiefs of Staff Instruction 3405.01, 2011; Nindl et al., 2018; Milley, 2016). We define soldier readiness based on the definitions above but adapt it to specifically refer to the impact of BH conditions.

For family readiness, we adopt DoD's definition (DoD Instruction 1342.22, 2012). A recent review of the literature addressing military family readiness identified 16 indicators of family readiness, including physical and mental health, social sup-

---

**Box 1.1 Definitions of Soldier and Family Readiness Used for the Project**

**Soldier Readiness:** The ability to perform mission-essential tasks and deploy without limitations from a BH condition.

**Family Readiness:** The state of being prepared to effectively navigate the challenges of daily living experienced in the unique context of military service, to include mobility and financial readiness, mobilization and deployment readiness, and personal and family life readiness.

port, couple functioning, children's functioning, parenting, finances and employment, deployment experiences, and accessibility of military services. Key findings of the review highlighted the importance of social, family, and marital support in promoting well-being and readiness (Hawkins et al., 2018). Another recent study on strengthening military family readiness noted the challenge of supporting today's increasingly complex and diverse family units that may include other members in addition to spouses and children, such as unmarried partners, siblings, and dependent elders (National Academies of Sciences, 2019). Although this DoD definition of family readiness could apply to children, adolescents, and the family as a whole, this report considered only adult family members who receive BH care.

The concept of readiness is complex, as indicated by the multiple and varied domains noted above related to soldier and family readiness. A key component of both soldier and family readiness is psychological well-being, which supports overall functioning (Lee et al., 2018; Trivedi et al., 2013). In civilian populations, assessment of functioning is traditionally focused on the degree of impairment or disability, if any, affecting self-care and daily activities, and is often related to current medical or mental health conditions. However, soldiers and adult family members tend to be relatively young and healthy, making measures of this type less useful in military populations. Our definition of soldier readiness highlights the importance of functioning in the context of the specific occupational tasks required to support the military mission. For adult family members, readiness involves functioning in the context of changes related to the soldier's potential absence, reintegration, and other circumstances specific to living in a military community. Although there is overlap in the domains included in both definitions of readiness (e.g., mental health, social functioning), each also may have unique domains (e.g., soldier physical fitness for military service, spouse's experiences during deployment). These differences present challenges to identifying a single metric that would aptly assess readiness for both soldiers and adult family members. In addition, family members (e.g., spouses, dependents) are increasingly accessing BH care at acute civilian medical facilities (Wooten et al., 2018), and there has been an increase in the overall net use of civilian care by spouses (and dependents) during soldier deployments (Larson et al., 2012). Any metric that the Army uses to monitor readiness would likely assess BH specialty care delivered at military treatment facilities (MTFs; i.e., direct care); therefore, its applicability to adult family members who use purchased care may be limited.

## Identifying Soldiers with Duty or Deployment Limitations

A core component of soldier readiness, as highlighted by our definition, is the ability to deploy. Soldiers who have a temporary or permanent medical condition that may render them not medically ready to deploy are put on a *profile*. In 2017, the Army issued a memorandum to standardize the application of profiles for BH conditions to appropriately inform commanders of duty limitations and related treatment support recommendations. The memorandum instructs health care providers to assess soldiers' medical readiness for duty during every clinical encounter. It also provides specific guidance on issuing profiles for specific BH conditions (e.g., severe psychiatric diagnoses) or treatments (e.g., inpatient BH care, selected psychotropic medications) and the minimum type of profile required (i.e., temporary or permanent) (U.S. Army, 2017). When a provider performs a clinical assessment and finds a soldier to be ready, but the soldier does not fully meet deployment criteria, the provider may issue a waiver. However, soldiers with BH waivers have been shown more likely than those without waivers to be medically evacuated from theater (Cronrath et al., 2017). The eProfile software application within the Medical Operational Data System (MODS) suite allows global tracking of soldiers who are on a profile.

Despite DoD's efforts to standardize the profiling process, Army providers have reported barriers to profiling, including the time required to write a profile, the impact of soldier restrictions on affected units, a lack of sufficient provider training in profiling, and the stigma associated with a profile, as well as a potential loss of confidentiality (Curley, Crouch, and Wilk, 2018). A recent study reconciled reported health care utilization and pharmacy data with documented profiles, and the results suggested that 1–3 percent of Army personnel without a profile met nondeployable criteria related to a BH or substance use condition (Curley and Warner, 2017). Interviews and focus groups with 29 Army BH providers revealed that there is also variation in how much and what particular information providers take into consideration when BH profiles are subsequently reviewed and soldiers are deemed ready or not ready to return to duty (Crouch et al., 2018).

## Monitoring and Improving the Quality of Behavioral Health Care

The monitoring of the quality of BH care is a multifaceted process. The learning BH system model—an extension of the learning health care system proposed by the Institute of Medicine in 2012—provides a framework and core strategies for delivering high-quality BH care (Stein, Adams, and Chambers, 2016). The model assumes that every health care system has areas that need improvement, and the core strategy to support continuous improvement is the transparent use of data. Core strategies include the routine use of data to understand variations in care that may inform quality improvement efforts and the monitoring of changes that result from those efforts. Systematic data collection provides an ongoing opportunity to mitigate these variations and continuously evaluate the effectiveness of care. Calculating performance rates for specific areas of care and subsequently sharing this information with health care providers and the public can create a learning environment that facilitates care improvement. DHA has shown its support for this model of monitoring quality. Its manual for clinical quality management in MHS describes the goal of clinical quality improvement through clinical measurement, knowledge sharing, and feedback (Defense Health Agency, 2019).

**Assessing the Quality of Behavioral Health Care**

When monitoring the quality of health care, three dimensions of care are commonly assessed: structure, process, and outcomes (Donabedian, 1988) (Figure 1.1). The structure of health care includes physical and organizational characteristics of care settings, such as facilities, equipment, personnel, and operational and financial administrative policies. Assessing aspects of structure informs whether a health care setting has the capacity to provide evidence-based care. The process of care includes activities related to the provision of care that is evidence based, including preventive care, diagnosis and treatment of health care problems, rehabilitation, and ongoing management of care. Care processes rely on adequate resources and mechanisms to support the delivery of evidence-based patient care. Optimal implementation can support improvements in care outcomes, such as patient symptoms, functioning, and satisfaction with care (also referred to as the patient experience of care). Consistent with a learning BH system, information about a health care system's performance across these three dimensions can reinforce areas of high performance and help identify areas of lower performance to inform ongoing quality improvement activities.

Ideally, outcome data that are collected for quality monitoring and improvement purposes (i.e., at the clinic, MTF, and organizational levels) should also be useful for providers in their work with individual patients. Individual patient outcomes (e.g., change in depression symptoms) provide clinicians with useful data to make timely decisions about treatment adjustments during the course of care, an approach called measurement-based care, that has shown improvement in patient outcomes (Harding et al., 2011; Slade et al., 2006).

Quality metrics[1] provide a means to evaluate the extent to which a recommended structural component, process of care, or outcome was achieved. Computed scores may be presented as a percentage of eligible facilities, encounters, or patients achieving the desired aspect of care (numerator) out of the total population of eligible facilities, encounters, or patients (denominator). A score can be compared with a desired target or benchmark. Examples of structural metrics include the percentage of MTFs that provide telehealth services for BH care or the average number of days' wait to receive

**Figure 1.1**
**Dimensions of Care**

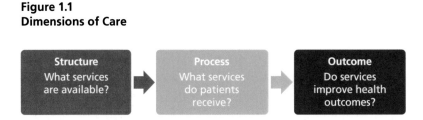

---

[1]   The standards used to assess quality of care are referred to as *quality measures, indicators,* or *metrics.* We use *quality metric* because that is the term that the Army has traditionally used.

specialty care for a new BH problem. An example of a process metric would be the percentage of patients with depression treated with an antidepressant who received at least 12 weeks of medication. A related outcome metric would be the percentage of patients with moderate to severe symptoms of depression, as measured by the Patient Health Questionnaire (PHQ-9; Spitzer et al., 1999) who had a clinically significant decrease in symptoms within 6 months. Note that while the underlying instrument (i.e., PHQ-9) provides a continuous depression symptom score, when information from this instrument is used in a quality metric, it is reported as a dichotomous metric (i.e., patient showed at least a clinically significant symptom improvement or not).

## Challenges of Implementing Quality Improvement

The implementation of a systemwide means to drive quality improvement, measure the success of that effort, and transparently use collected data to support identified strengths and target needed improvements can be challenging. Selected outcome metrics should reliably measure an outcome of interest, be related to associated processes of care, and be sensitive to changes in that care. When outcome metrics do not meet these standards, their use may lead to costly implementation programs that do not measure an outcome of interest and can cause institutional frustration at the lack of positive results (Martinez, Lewis, and Weiner, 2014). Therefore, outcome metrics should be selected carefully to meet a minimum standard of psychometric soundness.

Even when an appropriate outcome metric has been selected, an organization may find implementation burdensome. Metrics used to drive quality improvement have associated costs that need to be balanced with the potential gains that may be achieved. Implementation places a degree of burden on staff to administer and incorporate the quality metrics into the care provided. Those receiving care may also experience the burden of the time required to complete self-report measures, as well as some degree of fatigue when multiple self-report measurements are required.

In the face of these challenges, the Institute for Healthcare Improvement and other organizations have created tool kits to support the planning, launch, and management of successful quality improvement projects (see Institute for Healthcare Improvement, 2019b). In the United Kingdom, the National Health Service has created a tool to evaluate the potential for the success of quality improvement efforts that assesses several contextual factors that affect the viability of a program, such as data infrastructure, internal and external motivators, program staff skills, and organizational support (National Health Service, 2019). The Joint Commission, an independent certification organization for health care entities, has also issued guidance on the selection of sound outcome metrics for considering costs, implementation management challenges, and the use of data (The Joint Commission, undated). Therefore, the selection of an outcome metric for quality improvement is a decision that carries multiple implications for an organization and requires considering not only the psychometrics of the instrument of choice but also the organizational context in which it will be implemented.

## The Army's Efforts to Monitor and Improve Behavioral Health Care

The Army has instituted several efforts to ensure the delivery of high-quality, standardized BH care. These efforts have included centralizing workload management, consolidating BH provider services, creating satellite BH clinics within brigade work areas, and incorporating BH providers into primary care, as well as implementing processes for routine and periodic mental health screening and expanding services for family members (Hoge et al., 2015; Meadows et al., 2018). Although the military provides several support services to assist family members in managing the unique demands of living in the context of military service, family member participation in those services is voluntary (DoD Instruction 1342.22, 2012).

### Monitoring Quality of Behavioral Health Care

The Army uses structure, process, and outcome metrics to monitor the quality of BH care on an ongoing basis. Using data from the Behavioral Health Data Portal (BHDP; U.S. Army, 2016a), along with administrative encounter and pharmacy data from the MHS Data Repository (MHS, 2019), the Army can track multiple aspects of care. Figure 1.2 includes metrics specified in a 2018 DHA Procedural Instruction, which aimed to identify a standardized core set of BH treatment and outcome metrics (Defense Health Agency, 2018) that would be collected for DHA care delivered across all service branches.

**Figure 1.2**
**Metrics for Monitoring Specialty Care Behavioral Health Clinics**

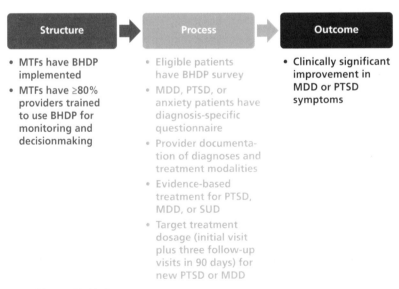

SOURCE: DHAPI, 2018.
NOTE: MDD = major depressive disorder; SUD = substance use disorder.

Routine symptom monitoring data are collected via BHDP from those receiving BH care in MTFs (direct care). BHDP focuses on symptom change in common BH conditions (e.g., PTSD, depression, anxiety disorders) during the course of treatment and provides essential information for clinicians to inform treatment management (DoD, 2016). These data also support ongoing evaluation of the effectiveness of Army's BH care and enable timely feedback about the impact of quality improvement efforts. However, symptom-based outcome metrics may not adequately capture whether soldiers who receive BH care are ready to perform the tasks required by their military occupational specialty (MOS) over the long term or whether family members who receive BH care can support them in doing so. Identifying how to most effectively measure readiness for soldiers and their families who receive BH care would allow the Army to optimize these outcomes.

**Expanding Outcome Monitoring to Include Readiness**
The Army's effectiveness relies on the readiness of its soldiers. In 2017 and based on existing definitions, 14 percent of active-component soldiers were classified as medically not ready (U.S. Army Public Health Center, 2018). The Army recently updated its policy on personnel readiness with modified medical deployability class definitions and set a targeted nondeployable rate of 5 percent or less (Secretary of the Army, 2018). To support the readiness of the force, the Army's Behavioral Health Service Line has instituted several strategies to promote readiness through effective BH care. As noted earlier, a soldier's medical readiness is assessed during every clinical encounter. At a minimum, this includes the soldier's mental status, risk of harm to self or others, symptom severity, prognosis for return to full duty, treatment needs, and risk of decompensation or further injury if the soldier participates in occupational activities (U.S. Army, 2017). Furthermore, the Army aims to provide timely access to high-quality BH care for both soldiers and their families.

Monitoring symptom improvement provides valuable information about the effectiveness of Army BH care and the proportion of patients whose symptoms improve. Yet these existing metrics do not fully capture whether soldiers and adult family members achieve readiness after receiving BH care. Incorporating one or more readiness metrics into its outcome monitoring program would allow the Army to expand their efforts to monitor and improve BH care. High quality BH care has the potential to improve multiple patient outcomes including psychiatric symptoms and functioning, such as improvements in occupational functioning (Lee et al., 2018; Trivedi et al., 2013). While soldier readiness could be viewed as a dichotomous concept (i.e., soldiers are either ready to deploy or not), our definition also includes "the ability to perform mission-essential tasks . . . without limitation from a BH condition." This definition highlights that soldier readiness can be viewed on a continuum and thus be measured continuously, similar to concepts like symptoms and functioning. As noted earlier, data collected for quality monitoring and improvement purposes should ideally be useful in the course of clinical care as well. Thus, considering instruments that assess readiness on a continuum could be particularly useful for both quality monitoring and clinical purposes.

## Organization of This Report

This report describes our efforts to identify potential metrics to assess readiness for soldiers and adult family members who receive BH care. While readiness to meet mission-related tasks, including deployment, is important for all soldiers and their families, this report focuses on the smaller population of soldiers and adult family members who receive BH care and the impact of that care on readiness. Additionally, while adult mental health has an impact on the well-being of other family members, this project does not address the readiness status of children, adolescents, or Army families as a whole. We aimed to identify outcome metrics that would assess readiness and contribute to monitoring the effectiveness of BH care.

In Chapter Two, we describe the methods used in our project. We conducted interviews with Army BH subject-matter experts and providers to document their perspectives on soldier and adult family readiness and its assessment. We also reviewed existing Army data sources that could be a source for readiness metrics and considered what new data collection could be of value. We searched the literature to identify instruments that could support a readiness metric for soldiers or adult family members, with an emphasis on those used in military populations. We also explored functioning metrics from core sets of BH outcome measures suggested by experts in the field. As noted earlier, there are potential costs and risks associated with implementing a metric that does not meet scientific standards (e.g., cost of data collection and reporting, lack of meaningful data, failure to capture patient improvement). Therefore, we developed rigorous criteria to evaluate potential readiness metrics.

Our findings are described in three chapters. In Chapter Three, we summarize respondents' perspectives on conceptual indicators of readiness, which allowed us to identify the most important concepts within the multidimensional concept of readiness that should be captured in a readiness metric. Relatedly, we also describe BH provider perspectives on assessing soldier readiness, such as the information that they integrate into their readiness assessments and how they decide whether to place a soldier on a profile. Chapter Four describes the results of our primary project objective, to identify metrics to assess readiness among soldiers and adult family members who receive BH care. Specifically, we describe our review of existing data sources and instruments and our application of our criteria to evaluate potential readiness metrics. As a supplement to our primary objective, we also documented BH expert and provider suggestions for strategies to improve readiness assessment, and these findings are described in Chapter Five. Chapter Six summarizes our findings and provides recommendations to help the Army identify optimal readiness metrics.

This report includes six appendixes that provide additional detail on, respectively, Army readiness policies, our interview protocols, the existing data sources that we identified, the search terms used in our instrument search, a summary of instruments identified in the literature, and a summary of instruments that we identified in a supplemental search.

CHAPTER TWO
# Methods

In this chapter, we describe the methods we used to identify potential metrics to assess readiness for soldiers and adult family members who receive BH care. We discuss the criteria that we used to evaluate potential readiness metrics and our approach to collecting and analyzing qualitative data from BH experts and providers on multiple aspects of readiness. In addition, we outline our review of existing MHS data sources that could serve as a basis for developing readiness metrics. Finally, we describe our process for identifying promising readiness metrics and instruments by searching the peer-reviewed literature on military personnel and their families and through area-expert recommendations.

## Criteria for Evaluating a Readiness Metric

As noted in Chapter One, it is important to implement only valid, reliable outcome metrics because of the significant costs associated with implementation. When metrics are not sufficiently vetted, the costs can be high, and implementation can have unintended consequences, such as the tracking of outcome results that are not valid. In this project, the focus of interest was the readiness of soldiers and adult family members receiving BH care. Therefore, a valid outcome metric's scores will be directly related to the BH care provided, allowing an evaluation of symptom improvement, the effectiveness of the care the patient received, and its impact on readiness.

We developed a set of criteria to use as a basis for evaluating the merits of candidate readiness metrics (Box 2.1). These criteria were adapted from those used by the National Quality Forum (NQF) to evaluate quality measures submitted for its potential endorsement (National Quality Forum, 2018). Characteristics of a desirable readiness metric include importance (the metric addresses a high-priority area in which performance could improve), feasibility (data exist to measure metric performance that are accessible without undue burden), scientific acceptability (the metric is reliable and valid in measuring the area of interest and sensitive to change), and usability (providers view the metric as useful and informative in assessing care). However, because this project was limited to identifying readiness metrics, the criteria do not include all

---

**Box 2.1 Criteria for Evaluating a Readiness Outcome Metric**

**Importance**
- Metric assesses a high-priority area in which there is an opportunity to improve

**Feasibility**
- Data to support the metric are retrievable without undue burden (e.g., existing data sources that are coded rather than unstructured, free text)
- Existing data or new metric data are collected routinely enough to capture changes that occurred while the soldier was receiving BH direct care
- Data can be accessed by Army BH leadership and/or DHA
- Metrics requiring new data collection should use instruments that are self-report, brief (30 or fewer items), and require no fee (e.g., no license fee or per administration fee)
- Data to support the metric must be linkable to soldiers and/or family members who receive Army BH direct care

**Scientific Acceptability**
- *Validity:* data are valid (assess soldier or family readiness as defined by the project)
- *Reliability:* data are reliable (data collection instrument consistently measures the outcome of interest)
- *Sensitivity to change:* data are sensitive to change (metric score would be expected to change if patient received high quality BH care)

**Usability**
- Readiness concept, as measured by the metric, is seen as valuable, important, and informative to providers in improving care

---

aspects of metric evaluation, such as field testing. Box 2.1 includes feasibility criteria that are important to the MHS in that they consider the costs of collecting existing or new data, prioritizing instruments that are brief, collect self-report data, and have no fee. The Joint Commission has emphasized the importance of using instruments with established psychometric properties (e.g., reliability, validity) (The Joint Commission, 2020). A selected instrument should be used routinely to establish norms and to ensure that care can be adjusted if needed. The instrument should be able to detect meaningful changes over time—that is, it should be sensitive to change beyond typical variation (The Joint Commission, 2020).

## Perspectives of Army Behavioral Health Experts and Behavioral Health Providers

As described in Chapter One, definitions of readiness, including those adopted for this project, are typically broad and multidimensional. Therefore, we sought stakeholder input to identify the most important aspects of readiness to aid our evaluation of potential readiness metrics that would be applicable in general and to those who received BH care. To obtain stakeholder perspectives on soldier and family readiness, we conducted interviews with Army BH subject-matter experts and Army BH providers.

### Interview Domains

Interviews with BH experts captured perspectives on (1) indicators of soldier and family readiness; (2) potential readiness metrics, including historical efforts to assess readiness, the value of existing data sources, and potential new data collection requirements; and (3) potential improvements to assessing readiness for soldiers and family members who receive BH care (Table 2.1). These interviews also allowed us to verify whether we had obtained copies of all policies related to readiness. See Appendix A for a list of relevant readiness policies.

BH provider interviews focused on (1) indicators of soldier and family readiness, (2) BH providers' approaches to assessing readiness, (3) interactions with commanders about BH care and force readiness, and (4) potential improvements to assessing readiness for soldiers and family members who receive BH care. Appendix B presents both interview protocols. We initially planned to interview Army unit commanders to document their perspectives on soldier readiness related to BH care. Unfortunately, scheduling conflicts prevented this, and the lack of commander input is a limitation of this study.

**Table 2.1**
**Domains of Behavioral Health Expert and Behavioral Health Provider Interviews**

| Domain | Army BH Experts | Army BH Providers |
|---|---|---|
| Indicators of readiness for soldiers and adult family members who have received BH care | X | X |
| Assessing readiness | | X |
| Interactions with commanders | | X |
| Metrics of readiness following BH care | X | |
| Improving readiness assessment | X | X |
| Readiness-related policies | X | |

**Eligibility Criteria and Recruitment**

Eligible Army BH experts included Army personnel who had participated in design- ing policies around readiness, assessed BH care quality or outcomes, been involved in designing systems that capture information to assess soldier or family readiness, or participated in BH quality monitoring and improvement activities.[1] The size of this eligible population is unknown, but we believe that there would be a relatively small number of Army personnel that would bring significant expertise in these areas. Army BH providers were eligible to participate if they delivered BH treatment to soldiers or family members at an Army MTF. Providers could have worked in a variety of BH set- tings, such as embedded behavioral health and BH specialty clinics. Eligible provider types included psychiatrists, psychologists, master's-level or advanced practice clini- cians, and counselors. The size of the eligible population is relatively large. A RAND study found that in 2016 the Army had 2,365 BH providers that were psychiatrists, psychiatric nurse practitioners, doctoral-level psychologists, or master's-level clinicians (i.e., psychologists, social workers) (Hepner et al., 2017).

We recruited BH experts and providers in collaboration with the Army, which provided a list of 20 potential BH experts. We agreed with the recommended partici- pant selection, and Army BH leadership emailed potential respondents to notify them of the study. Subsequently, we scheduled telephone or in-person interviews, which were conducted between March and May 2019. For BH provider interviewees, Army BH leadership recommended a small number of Army installations, from which we selected two for interviews. Army BH leaders connected us with the director of psy- chological health at each installation, each of whom identified potential participants and provided us with an interview schedule. The interviews were conducted either in person or by phone in March and May 2019. For both BH experts and provid- ers, participation was optional; installation directors of BH were tasked with identify- ing potential BH provider participants, which may have introduced some bias in the perspectives we documented (e.g., identifying providers who were more interested in readiness issues or policies).

**Analytic Approach**

Interviews were conducted by two researchers, ensuring that one person was able to take detailed notes, as interviews were not recorded. Notes from the interviews were checked for quality, completeness, and accuracy by both the interviewer and notetaker assigned to each interview. To summarize perspectives for each interview domain, the project team used qualitative methods, incorporating Rapid and Rigorous Qualita- tive Data Analysis (RADaR) (Watkins, 2017) and Qualitative Description (Bradshaw,

---

[1]  Due to regulatory requirements, we planned for BH experts and BH providers to be primarily active duty or DoD government civilians but allowed up to nine contractors in each group. Ultimately, no contractors participated.

Atkinson, and Doody, 2017; Neergaard et al., 2009) techniques. The RADaR technique uses an expedited and team-oriented approach for organizing and analyzing interview data, which supported the project's rapid timeline. The Qualitative Description approach is particularly useful where information is required directly from those experiencing the phenomenon under investigation and where time and resources are limited. Qualitative Description uses a structured interview guide with open-ended questions to gather the information directly from those with relevant, firsthand experience, such as BH providers assessing soldier readiness. By using this approach, we could capture and explore in detail the perspectives of the participants.

The detailed interview notes were entered into a spreadsheet, organized by interview prompt and interview identification code. A researcher examined the responses across respondent type (i.e., BH expert vs. BH provider) and presented a list of topics organized by prompt to the research team. Following team discussion, final topics were coded using a count (1/0) to represent the presence or absence of the topic. Next, the team reviewed the summary topics and proposed themes (i.e., individual topics grouped into themes). We summed counts and computed a percentage for each topic and theme. Percentages were calculated using the sum of the counts divided by number of respondents who provided a response to the relevant prompt.

## Respondent Characteristics

We interviewed 18 BH experts and 24 BH providers (Table 2.2). Most BH experts were active duty, while the majority of BH providers were Army civilians. Approximately a third of BH providers were active duty; three were also part of the U.S. Army Forces Command (FORSCOM). Among active-duty participants, BH experts tended to be higher ranked than BH providers. BH experts were more likely to have both a clinical and administrative role, while BH providers were more likely to only have a clinical role. Participants were practicing across a variety of clinical settings, with BH experts most likely to be practicing in a multidisciplinary outpatient BH clinic and most BH providers practicing in an embedded BH clinic. Half of the BH experts were psychiatrists, and two-thirds of BH providers were licensed clinical social workers or psychologists.

While we aimed to collect information about soldier and family readiness, no providers reported currently providing direct clinical services to adult family members. This may reflect that many or most adult family members receive BH care from purchased care providers. Alternatively, it may be an artifact of the providers who were selected by the directors of psychological health at the individual installations or the small number of providers whom we interviewed. Those who saw patients through the Army's Child and Family Behavioral Health Services (CAFBHS) clinics saw children. Respondents who felt that they had adequate prior experience treating families or who were familiar with family member policies opted to respond to interview questions related to family readiness. Thus, the resulting sample limited our ability to capture

**Table 2.2**
**Army Behavioral Health Experts and Behavioral Health Providers Interviewed**

| Characteristics | Army BH Experts (*N* = 18) | Army BH Providers (*N* = 24) |
|---|---|---|
| **Status** | | |
| Active duty | 13 | 8 |
| Army civilian | 5 | 16 |
| **Rank** | | |
| Colonel | 4 | 0 |
| Lieutenant colonel | 8 | 2 |
| Major | 1 | 4 |
| Captain | 0 | 2 |
| **Role** | | |
| Clinical | 0 | 16 |
| Administrative | 4 | 0 |
| Both | 14 | 8 |
| **Location of current clinical activities[a]** | | |
| CAFBHS | 2 | 3 |
| Embedded BH clinic | 0 | 15 |
| Inpatient/residential | 4 | 2 |
| Intensive outpatient program | 1 | 0 |
| Multidisciplinary outpatient BH | 8 | 3 |
| Primary care | 1 | 0 |
| Soldier Family Care Center | 0 | 1 |
| SUD Clinical Care (SUDCC) | 0 | 2 |
| No current clinical activities | 3 | 0 |
| **Provider type** | | |
| Licensed clinical social worker | 4 | 9 |
| Master's-level counselor | 0 | 1 |
| Physician assistant | 1 | 0 |
| Psychiatric advanced practice nurse | 0 | 3 |
| Psychiatrist | 9 | 3 |
| Psychologist | 4 | 7 |
| SUDCC/Army Substance Abuse Program counselor | 0 | 1 |

[a] Individuals may be included in more than one category.

perspectives on family readiness. In addition, some respondents declined to respond to a few questions: Two BH providers did not currently treat soldiers and declined to provide responses about assessing soldier readiness and putting a soldier on a profile, and six BH providers declined to respond to the prompt about indicators of family readiness because they were not currently treating family members.

## Review of Existing Data Sources

We reviewed existing data sources that could potentially support a readiness metric for soldiers and/or adult family members. The primary advantage of using an existing data source is that the additional effort and cost associated with relying on these data may be minimal. Still, because existing data sources were not designed with the explicit purpose of supporting a readiness metric, we anticipated that we would need to evaluate the limitations of these data sources carefully.

Using information available from published sources (e.g., websites) and perspectives provided during interviews with BH experts and providers, we identified 15 potential data sources (listed in Appendix C). We did not include data sources that were limited to a specific program or service (e.g., Family Advocacy Program, Army Community Services) or to a limited population (e.g., Drug and Alcohol Management Information System). For each source we considered, we evaluated the appropriateness of variables contained within the source for potential use in a readiness metric (to the extent that we had visibility of specific data elements). The criteria we used to evaluate the data elements in each source included those listed in Box 2.1 as well as the population to whom the data applied (e.g., data sources covering only reservists were excluded). Data sources that met these inclusion criteria were further studied for their potential use in constructing a readiness metric.

## Search of the Literature to Identify Instruments for Readiness Metrics

### Search Strategy

We conducted a search of the literature to identify instruments that have been used to assess the readiness of soldiers or adult family members. While there are many components that affect readiness (e.g., social support, financial constraints, family issues, mental and physical health), we aimed to ultimately identify a single instrument that would support a readiness metric that would assess multiple components of readiness. The review focused on instruments that captured the unique demands on soldiers and their families and their impact on readiness.

We executed two separate searches of the peer-reviewed literature, one for military personnel and one for military families. We searched the title, abstract, subject heading, and keywords in Academic Search Complete, PsycINFO, PubMed, and Web of Science from 2008 to 2018 for the following terms (see Appendix D for a complete list of the search terms):

- military personnel or military family or military spouse
- and a metric, measure, survey, instrument, profile, or screening tool
- and readiness
- and a component that affects readiness (e.g., mental functioning, behavioral health, well-being).

The searches yielded a combined total of 171 articles. We reviewed titles and abstracts of the 171 articles for inclusion of a measure, outcome metric, or indicator of readiness (or proxy of readiness), an adult population, and published in English. We excluded articles if they focused only on a symptom measure that was not used as a measure of readiness, the studied population was under the age of 18, or the instrument was a military-unit measure rather than an individual measure. Out of the 171 articles, 56 were retained for full text review. Most of the articles were excluded during the title and abstract phase because they did not include an instrument that would support a readiness metric.

**Full Text Review**
The 56 articles that moved to full text review were screened a second time using the same inclusion and exclusion criteria as the title and abstract screening to confirm the inclusion of an instrument that would support a readiness metric. As a result, we retained 14 articles that included a total of 50 instruments. (See Appendix E for the complete list of instruments.) Reasons for article exclusion included a lack of a readiness component, a focus solely on a military-unit-level measurement (not a metric of the individual), or a focus on condition-specific symptoms.

From the 14 remaining articles, we extracted the following data: instrument name, instrument source, readiness domain, population studied, typical setting of use, timing of administration, number of instrument items, length of administration time, reliability, validity, predictive validity, and sensitivity to change. The extracted data were reviewed, and the metrics were evaluated by the research team to explore their feasibility and application for soldiers and adult family members who received BH care. To remain in consideration, a metric needed to be self-report, contain no more than 30 items, and assess readiness/functioning. Instruments that were limited to a subcomponent affecting readiness (e.g., social support) or past events (e.g., history of past stressors) were excluded.

**Supplemental Search for Instruments for Readiness Metrics**

In addition to the formal search of the literature for instruments, we identified instruments measuring functioning recommended in core sets of BH outcome instruments and other metrics suggested by BH experts. (See Appendix F for a full list of instruments from the supplemental search.) The purpose of the supplemental review was to complement our identification of potential instruments addressing functioning from the literature with those that have been recommended for this purpose for general use. Similar criteria as described above for the instrument search were used to evaluate the metrics from the supplemental search to select candidate metrics for continuing consideration.

# CHAPTER THREE

# Measuring the Readiness of Soldiers and Families

In this chapter, we describe the perspectives of BH experts and BH providers on conceptual indicators of readiness. These perspectives provided important information about which aspects of readiness should be captured in a readiness metric. Although data for a readiness metric could come from a variety of sources (e.g., existing databases, patient self-report instrument), BH providers play an important role in assessing readiness within BH settings. Thus, we also summarize findings from our qualitative interviews with BH providers on topics related to assessing soldier readiness, communicating with commanders, and deciding whether to put a soldier on a profile. Not surprisingly, respondents covered many of the same topics here that they discussed with conceptual indicators of readiness.

## Conceptual Indicators of Readiness

As noted in Chapter One, we define soldier readiness as "the ability to perform mission-essential tasks and deploy without limitations from a BH condition." Family readiness was defined as "the state of being prepared to effectively navigate the challenges of daily living experienced in the unique context of military service, to include mobility and financial readiness, mobilization and deployment readiness, and personal and family life readiness." We asked BH experts and providers whether they had any concerns about these definitions, and none voiced a concern.

### Indicators of Soldier Readiness

We asked BH experts ($N = 18$) and providers ($N = 24$) what indicators they observed that suggested that soldiers were *not ready*. The indicators of lack of soldier readiness could be grouped in four categories:

- psychiatric symptoms/diagnoses
- being on a profile
- psychiatric treatment
- impaired functioning.

It should be noted that these categories are highly related from a clinical perspective and, thus, their occurrence is likely highly correlated within a soldier.

Psychiatric symptoms or diagnoses were frequently mentioned by both BH experts and providers (BH experts, $n$ = 12; BH providers, $n$ = 22). For example, more than half of respondents mentioned that a psychiatric diagnosis, such as MDD and PTSD, indicated that a soldier was not ready (BH experts, $n$ = 11; BH providers, $n$ = 15). And approximately one-fourth mentioned severe mental illness and approximately one-fourth mentioned the presence of safety concerns—namely, suicidal or homicidal ideation—as indicators that a soldier was not ready (in both cases, BH experts, $n$ = 4; BH providers, $n$ = 6). Nearly as many respondents noted that alcohol or drug use often indicates lack of readiness (BH experts, $n$ = 5; BH providers, $n$ = 4). BH providers were more likely than BH experts were to report that high scores on BH symptom screening measures or more severe BH symptoms noted during the clinical interview would be indicators that a soldier was not ready (BH experts, $n$ = 1; BH providers, $n$ = 7).

These responses were largely consistent with and likely influenced by existing policy guidance on applying profiles. The Minimum Profile Guidance instructs providers when to apply a temporary profile related to psychiatric symptoms (e.g., suicidal ideation) (U.S. Army, 2016b) or psychiatric diagnoses (e.g., SUD) (U.S. Army, 2017; DoD Instruction 6490.07, 2010). Overall, about one-fifth of respondents indicated that a soldier's already being on a profile would indicate that a soldier is *not ready* (BH experts, $n$ = 5; BH providers, $n$ = 4).[1]

Respondents also frequently reported that aspects of psychiatric treatment were indicators of a lack of readiness (BH experts, $n$ = 11; BH providers, $n$ = 12). For example, over half of BH experts and nearly half of BH providers reported that frequent use of BH care suggested that a soldier may not be ready (BH experts, $n$ = 11; BH providers, $n$ = 11). Some respondents also noted that psychotropic medication treatment, such as being on a medication that restricted deployment or a newly prescribed medication, would also be indicators of lack of readiness (BH experts, $n$ = 3; BH providers, $n$ = 4). These responses also align with existing policy, which instructs providers in how to apply a temporary profile regarding psychotropic medication use (MEDCOM Policy Memo 17-079, 2017; DoD Instruction 6490.07, 2010).

The final theme reported by respondents was impaired functioning, including both occupational (BH experts, $n$ = 7; BH providers, $n$ = 20) and social functioning (BH experts, $n$ = 10; BH providers, $n$ = 15). Related to occupational functioning, two-thirds of BH providers reported poor job performance or poor relationships with superiors as important indicators of a lack of readiness (BH providers, $n$ = 16); a lower proportion of BH experts endorsed these factors (BH experts, $n$ = 7). Fewer respondents

---

[1]  Fewer respondents may have mentioned this because it was not included as a follow-up probe in our interview guide. Alternatively, respondents may have viewed being on a profile as an administrative process that follows after a soldier is determined to be not ready rather than a presenting characteristic of the soldier.

noted that administrative actions or disciplinary events indicated a lack of readiness (BH experts, $n = 2$; BH providers, $n = 6$).

Difficulties with social functioning was another prominent theme that was frequently mentioned by both BH experts and providers. For example, half of BH experts and nearly half of BH providers noted that the presence of family stressors or other family problems were indicators of lack of readiness (BH experts, $n = 9$; BH providers, $n = 10$). Some respondents also mentioned reduced social cohesion or inability to work in a team (BH experts, $n = 3$; BH providers, $n = 8$) and soldier immaturity, such as not understanding the level of responsibility and dedication required to be a soldier, as indicators of lack of readiness (BH experts, $n = 1$; BH providers, $n = 4$).

### Indicators of Readiness for Adult Family Members

We also asked BH experts and providers what indicators they had observed to suggest that adult family members are not ready. The indicators related to lack of readiness for adult family members were similar to those noted for soldiers:

- impaired functioning
- psychiatric symptoms/diagnoses
- psychiatric treatment.

One-third of BH providers declined to respond to this question, as they did not believe that they had adequate clinical experience with this population, so the following findings include the 18 BH providers who provided a response. Indicators of lack of readiness fell into three categories: impaired functioning, psychiatric symptoms/diagnoses, and psychiatric treatment. Aspects of functioning defined the most common theme; half of respondents highlighted impaired overall or general functioning (BH experts, $n = 12$; BH providers, $n = 10$), whereas fewer reported that impaired social (BH experts, $n = 4$; BH providers, $n = 4$) or occupational functioning (BH experts, $n = 2$; BH providers, $n = 1$) were indicators of a lack of readiness. For example, half of BH experts and one-third of BH providers noted that if the adult family member cannot function independently (without the soldier), that would indicate that the adult family member is not ready (BH experts, $n = 10$; BH providers, $n = 6$). Other aspects of overall functioning mentioned by respondents included the presence of family stressors, lack of childcare, involvement with the Family Advocacy Program or the Exceptional Family Member Program, and inability to function outside the United States. A few noted that if a family member is not well, then a soldier is not well.

Some respondents highlighted other aspects of impaired social or occupational functioning in their responses. For example, about one-fifth of respondents reported that marital or personal relationship stressors were indicators of lack of readiness (BH experts, $n = 3$; BH providers, $n = 4$). Only a few respondents noted that problems with occupational functioning, such as challenges at a job or finding employment, suggested that an adult family member was not ready (BH experts, $n = 2$; BH providers, $n = 1$).

The second theme was the presence of psychiatric symptoms or diagnoses, mentioned more frequently by BH experts than by BH providers (BH experts, $n = 8$; BH providers, $n = 2$). For example, about one-fifth of BH experts mentioned mental health issues (BH experts, $n = 4$), and about one-fifth mentioned alcohol and drug issues (BH experts, $n = 4$), while far fewer BH providers mentioned these (BH providers, $n = 2$ and $n = 0$, respectively). The final theme identified, psychiatric treatment, was mentioned only by BH experts ($n = 3$). Specifically, they reported that high utilization of behavioral health care by a family member suggested that the family member was *not ready*.

## Provider Approaches to Assessing Soldier Readiness

During our interviews with BH providers, we asked providers to elaborate on how they approach assessing the readiness of soldiers. Specifically, we asked about the type of information BH providers find informative in assessing soldier readiness, their collaboration with commanders, and how they decide whether to place a soldier on a profile.

### Information Behavioral Health Providers Use to Assess Soldier Readiness

BH providers were asked about the information that they incorporate into their assessments of readiness for soldiers who receive BH care. Two providers declined to respond to this question (a child psychiatrist and child psychologist who did not routinely assess soldier readiness), giving us a total of 22 respondents. BH providers reported using a variety of information to assess soldier readiness, which we categorized according to six themes:

- patient self-report measures
- clinical interviews
- collateral information
- occupational functioning
- current and past BH treatment
- policy guidance.

The two types of information mentioned most frequently were patient self-report measures ($n = 19$) and clinical interviews ($n = 20$). Most BH providers reported that they used patient self-report measures that were typically collected in BHDP. The clinical interview is a semi-structured or unstructured approach clinicians use to assess the patient's clinical presentation (e.g., symptoms, diagnoses, history, psychosocial factors) and inform the treatment plan. Most providers specifically mentioned the clinical interview ($n = 18$) as a key approach to assess soldier symptomatology and inform diagnosis. Some providers specifically mentioned aspects of the clinical interview, including assessing for risk issues (e.g., suicide risk) ($n$ = 3), alcohol and drug use ($n$ = 5), and consistency between self-report measures and the clinical interview ($n$ = 2). BH providers frequently reported also integrating collateral information in their assessment of readiness ($n$ = 17). For example, nearly three-quarters of providers ($n$ = 16) reported consulting with command to integrate their perspective on occupational or risk issues that the soldier may be experiencing. Fewer reported integrating information from family ($n$ = 9) or peers ($n$ = 4). Relatedly, some providers noted that they also consider information from a variety of sources about the soldier's occupational functioning ($n$ = 5), such as whether the soldier is ready to deploy ($n$ = 3) or assessment of job performance ($n$ = 4).

Several BH providers noted that they integrate a review of current and past BH treatment ($n$ = 9), typically through a review of the medical record. Specifically, one-third of providers ($n$ = 7) mentioned reviewing treatment history. Individual providers also noted various aspects of treatment including inpatient treatment, stability on medication, and length of time in BH care. Finally, a few providers noted that they refer to policy guidance ($n$ = 5), such as existing regulations ($n$ = 4) or the Behavioral Health Readiness Evaluation and Decisionmaking Instrument (B-REDI) tool ($n$ = 1). B-REDI is a decision support tool designed to help providers determine whether to write a profile for a soldier for a BH condition.

The ability to perform duties without limitations is central to soldier readiness. We asked BH providers whether they assessed the *specific duties* that soldiers needed to perform as part of their readiness assessment (23 respondents). Most providers relied on the soldier's MOS ($n$ = 17) and/or the soldier's description of specific duties ($n$ = 18) in making their readiness assessment. Some providers noted that the MOS is quite general and may not accurately capture what the soldier needs to be able to do. About three-quarters of providers ($n$ = 18) reported they communicate with command to assess the specific duties that a soldier must be ready to perform. The small proportion of providers that did not routinely assess specific duties focused rather on clinical diagnoses or believed that specific duties were not relevant to addressing the central question of whether a soldier could deploy.

### Behavioral Health Providers' Collaboration with Commanders

When asked if their view of readiness is different from that of commanders, three-quarters of providers ($n$ = 18) indicated there were differences in perspectives. The most frequent reason provided for the differences was that BH providers and commanders have different roles and priorities ($n$ = 9). For example, commanders rely on soldiers to be ready to fulfill the mission, and meeting BH needs may be associated with a soldier's not being ready. Another frequent reason reported was that soldiers may present differently in different situations ($n$ = 7), hiding or exaggerating symptoms with their commander or a BH provider. For example, soldiers may attempt to hide psychiatric symptoms from their commander, perhaps due to stigma or career implications, or may show more symptoms to avoid being deployed. Providers also mentioned that they have sometimes felt pressure from command to change their assessment of a soldier ($n = 6$) and have had instances where their decision about a soldier's readiness was "overruled" by command ($n = 6$) (e.g., taking a soldier on a deployment when the provider assessed the soldier as not ready).

**Behavioral Health Provider Decision to Place Soldier on a Profile**
BH providers were asked what influences whether they put a soldier on a profile. Two providers who were not seeing soldiers declined to respond to this question, leaving 22 respondents. There were several similarities in the information sources that providers draw on to assess readiness (described earlier) and what influences their decision to place a soldier on a profile. Five themes emerged:

- psychiatric symptoms/diagnoses
- psychiatric treatment
- collateral information
- occupational functioning
- policy guidance.

Psychiatric symptoms and diagnoses were the most frequent factor that influenced whether a provider placed a soldier on a profile ($n = 20$). For example, nearly two-thirds of providers ($n = 15$) considered risk/safety issues (e.g., suicide risk) and half broadly referred to psychiatric symptoms or diagnoses ($n = 12$). Aspects of psychiatric treatment ($n = 10$) also influenced these decisions, with amount of BH utilization, including whether psychiatric hospitalization was needed ($n = 7$), use of specific psychotropic medications ($n = 5$), and level of response to treatment ($n = 1$) as significant factors. One-third ($n = 8$) reported that communication with command about occupational functioning or symptom presentation was a factor in their decisionmaking. Level of occupational functioning was mentioned by several providers ($n = 10$), including deployability ($n = 6$), performance of duties ($n = 5$) (e.g., ability to complete assignments), ability to support the mission ($n = 3$), and presence of any duty limitations ($n = 2$) (e.g., limited duties due to medical limitations). Lastly, about a third of providers ($n = 7$) mentioned that policy guidance influences their decision to place a soldier on a profile. For example, providers reported that they refer to Army retention standards ($n = 1$), deployment standards and guidelines ($n = 4$), or B-REDI ($n = 3$). Although providers were asked if time pressure or competing demands influenced their assessment of whether to place a soldier on a profile, none of the providers endorsed this as a factor. Not surprisingly and as noted earlier, the factors mentioned that influence whether a provider places a soldier on a profile align with current policy guidance.

In addition to reporting what influences their decision to place a soldier on a profile, some providers shared their perspective on whether their decision to apply a profile varies based on the type of profile (e.g., temporary vs. permanent). The examples often aligned with the themes discussed above. For example, if a soldier is completing a course of treatment and this information needs to be communicated to command, a provider will apply a temporary profile. Other reasons included the soldier's receiving treatment in SUDCC, which aligns with policy (DoD Instruction 6490.07, 2010), or concerns about the soldier's ability to perform during field training. Providers also mentioned that if they apply a permanent profile, it often requires approval by their superior, and the soldier is typically sent to the Medical Review Board once the permanent profile is applied. Respondents also mentioned they would apply a permanent profile if a soldier did not improve following a temporary profile or had a chronic condition that prevented them from having a successful experience in the Army.

## Summary

In this chapter, we described the conceptual indicators of soldier and adult family readiness identified by BH experts and providers. For soldiers, the indicators can be grouped into four categories: psychiatric symptoms/diagnoses, being on a profile, psychiatric treatment, and impaired functioning. Indicators for adult family member were similar and included impaired functioning, psychiatric symptoms/diagnoses, and psychiatric treatment. These findings highlight the multidimensional nature of readiness and the factors that affect it for both soldiers and their families. Both BH experts and providers identified psychiatric symptoms or diagnoses as prominent indicators of lack of readiness, with this theme being mentioned more frequently regarding soldiers than families. These results suggest that these stakeholders find that BH symptoms are an important indicator of readiness, which provides support for the Army's ongoing efforts to track symptom-based BH outcome measures. Another indicator of readiness mentioned for soldiers related to the receipt of psychiatric treatment. Specific diagnoses and treatments are included in the guidance for placing a soldier on a BH profile, so it was not unexpected that this guidance was reflected in what respondents identified as indicators of lack of readiness. Relatedly, some respondents mentioned that already being on a profile indicated that the soldier was not ready.

Notably, the findings also highlight the significant role of multiple aspects of functioning, including occupational functioning (particularly for soldiers), social functioning, and general functioning (particularly for family members) related to readiness. The Army's current efforts to monitor outcomes for soldiers and adult family members who receive BH care do not include outcome metrics that assess functioning. These results suggest that including functioning may provide a more complete assessment of both soldier and family readiness.

Although data for a readiness metric could come from a variety of sources, BH providers routinely assess readiness in their clinical practice. We also described interview findings related to the information BH providers use to assess soldier readiness, whether BH providers' view of readiness was different from that of commanders, and how BH providers decide whether to place a soldier on a profile.

BH providers use a variety of information to make a readiness assessment, including patient self-report measures, a clinical interview, collateral information obtained primarily from commanders, assessment of the soldier's occupational functioning, current and past BH treatment, and policy guidance. Providers also reported that as part of their readiness assessment, they consider the specific duties that soldiers must be able to perform, which may be evident by the soldier's MOS or may require a soldier's description of his or her responsibilities. When we asked BH providers whether their view of readiness differed from that of commanders, most said that there were differences in perspective, owing primarily to their different roles and priorities, as well as differences in how the soldier presents to a commander and to a BH provider. Finally, when providers are deciding whether to place a soldier on a profile, they base the decision on the soldier's psychiatric symptoms, diagnoses, related treatment, collateral information, occupational functioning, and policy guidance. Some providers reported that they most often applied temporary profiles, but some assigned a permanent profile for chronic conditions, if the soldier required a disability evaluation, or if the soldier did not improve after being on a temporary profile.

# CHAPTER FOUR

# Evaluation of Existing Data Sources and Potential Instruments to Support a Readiness Metric

In this chapter, we describe the results of our evaluation of potential data sources and instruments that could be utilized for a readiness metric. Specifically, we present the results of our evaluation of existing data sources, followed by an evaluation of potential patient self-report instruments to support monitoring readiness.

## Evaluation of Existing Data Sources

We reviewed existing data sources to determine whether data elements that are currently collected and housed in military data systems could support a soldier or family member readiness metric. Using the criteria described in Chapter Two, we considered the content of each data source (to the extent possible) and its direct applicability to measuring readiness. Based on this evaluation, we subsequently narrowed these down from 15 data sources to two promising sources (Table 4.1): BHDP and eProfile (Hoge et al., 2015; Womak Army Medical Center, undated). The complete list of data sources that we considered, along with a description of each and a brief explanation of why we excluded a source from our full evaluation, can be found in Appendix C. The primary reasons for excluding a data source were that the data elements were collected too infrequently (e.g., annually), limited to a specific population (e.g., reservists), or did not address readiness (e.g., personnel files).

**Table 4.1**
**Existing Data Sources Evaluated for Supporting a Readiness Metric**

| Data Source | Description |
|---|---|
| BHDP | Module within MODS designed to track BH symptoms to inform treatment and improve BH care |
| eProfile | Tracks soldiers who have been identified as having a permanent or temporary medical condition that may result in medical nonreadiness for deployment |

## Evaluation of the Behavioral Health Data Portal for Potential Source of Readiness Data

BHDP is an online system used in MTFs (i.e., direct care) that contains patient-reported symptom data and clinician-reported information about BH treatment frequency and modalities (U.S. Army, 2016a). The goals of BHDP are to improve BH clinical care and risk tracking (e.g., suicide risk), to support the evidence-based use of outcome data to assess responses to BH care, and to integrate relevant sources of data to help improve coordination of care. BHDP includes several self-report instruments that assess psychiatric symptoms (e.g., PTSD, depression, anxiety, insomnia, suicide risk) and related concepts (e.g., general distress).

### Experts' Perspectives on the Behavioral Health Data Portal

The use of existing data sources to support a readiness metric was a topic addressed during our interviews with BH experts. When asked about existing data sources that could support a readiness metric, more than three-quarters of the BH experts ($n$ = 14) suggested BHDP, as it is the current vehicle for collecting data from adult patients (e.g., soldiers, adult family members) who are receiving BH treatment in MTFs (i.e., direct care). Although some respondents suggested using BHDP instruments to monitor readiness, most of these instruments do not measure readiness directly. Rather, they assess conditions that can affect readiness (e.g., suicidality, depression, insomnia, general distress, alcohol use) and inform BH treatment. On the other hand, some respondents voiced concerns about BHDP as a practical tool, citing the need for more computers and better maintenance to reduce downtime and slow performance. BHDP can be informative for the provider, but it can be a source of frustration for the soldier who may feel burdened by the need to complete multiple questionnaires. Therefore, any proposed metric should be as parsimonious as possible.

### Walter Reed Functional Impairment Scale

While most of the instruments in BHDP assess symptomology that may affect readiness and inform treatment, they do not address the broader construct of readiness. However, we determined that the Walter Reed Functional Impairment Scale (WRFIS) within BHDP is a promising instrument for supporting a readiness metric as it addresses several aspects of functioning.[1] The WRFIS was also suggested as a readiness metric by two of the BH expert interview respondents. The content of the WRFIS is summarized in Table 4.2.

The original WRFIS is a 14-item self-report questionnaire focused on physical, occupational, social, and personal functional limitations, with responses to each question about difficulty performing functions using a five-point scale (no difficulty at all, a little difficulty, moderate difficulty, quite a bit of difficulty, and extreme dif-

---

[1]  The WRFIS was mentioned as a potential instrument during stakeholder interviews. It was not detected in our instrument search because the term *readiness* is not associated or linked to the publication.

**Table 4.2**
**Content of 14-Item and 6-Item Walter Reed Functional Impairment Scale**

| WRFIS Item | 14-Item | 6-Item |
|---|---|---|
| How much **difficulty** do you have with the following? | | |
| *Physical functioning* | | |
| Your ability to do PT or exercise | | |
| (PT = physical training to maintain fitness required for military service) | X | X |
| Your ability to carry heavy loads | X | |
| *Occupational functioning* | | |
| Your overall work performance | X | X |
| The accuracy of your work[a] | X | |
| The quality of your work[a] | X | |
| Your ability to complete assigned tasks | X | |
| Your ability to multitask | X | |
| Your problem-solving at work | X | |
| *Social functioning* | | |
| Your ability to get along with your coworkers | X | X |
| Your ability to interact with social groups (e.g., church, sports, clubs) | X | |
| Your ability to get along with family or friends | X | X |
| Your ability to have a close relationship (e.g., spouse, girlfriend/boyfriend) | X | X |
| *Personal functioning* | | |
| Your ability to handle personal responsibilities (e.g., maintaining the car, keeping appointments, running errands) | X | X |
| Your ability to get your bills paid on time | X | |

[a] BHDP currently includes the 6-item WRFIS plus these additional items.

ficulty). The WRFIS has a score range of 14–70. Many commonly used instruments that measure functioning address limitations based on physical or mental conditions and are intended to assess functioning in adults and elderly populations with varying levels of health or chronic disease burden. The WRFIS, on the other hand, was developed specifically for use with active-duty military personnel, a population that faces unique occupational physical demands and opportunities for exposure to stressful events (Herrell et al., 2014). The WRFIS assesses four domains of functioning: physical (ability to do physical training and carry heavy loads); occupational (overall work performance, accuracy of work, quality of work, ability to complete assigned tasks, ability to multitask, and problem solving at work); social (ability to get along with coworkers, ability to interact with social groups, ability to get along with family and friends, and ability to have a close relationship [e.g., spouse, girlfriend/boyfriend]), and personal (e.g., ability to handle personal responsibilities, ability to get bills paid on time).

Using a cross-sectional sample of soldiers who had recently returned from deployment ($n$ = 3,380), the instrument's developers showed that greater impairment as measured by the 14-item WRFIS was strongly associated with a worse perception of overall health, more absenteeism, and higher health care utilization (Herrell et al., 2014). When computing score quartiles, they noted that the percentage of participants meeting criteria for major depression or PTSD was less than 4.5 percent among those below the median level of impairment and greater than 30 percent among those in the highest quartile of impairment. Higher WRFIS scores were also correlated with negative occupational and social performance outcomes, such as concerns expressed by the soldier's supervisor or receiving corrective training. Quartile score boundaries for the 14-item version were 14–15 indicating no difficulty or impairment, 16–19 indicating little impairment, 20–26 indicating moderate impairment, and 27–70 indicating extreme impairment. Internal consistency reliability was high (Cronbach's $\alpha$ = 0.92).

A shorter, six-item version of the WRFIS has also been developed, with a score range of 6–30. The WRFIS that is currently in BHDP contains eight items: the same six items as the shorter WRFIS, plus an additional two items related to occupational function. Both short versions address the same four domains of functioning as the longer version. In a study of soldier perceptions of integration into a new unit, researchers measured various soldier characteristics, including depression and anxiety symptoms and functional impairment. Functional impairment was measured using the six-item WRFIS. The results indicated that a positive perception of personal integration was significantly associated with fewer mental health symptoms, fewer anger reactions, better unit climate, and less functional impairment (Adrian et al., 2018).

Both the original and six-item versions of the WRFIS were undergoing further development and testing at the time of this writing, including validation against the Veterans RAND 12-Item Health Survey (VR-12) (Spiro et al., 2004), and the results were not yet published (Duffy, 2019). To date, no studies have examined the WRFIS's sensitivity to change.

Because the WRFIS targets occupational functioning, along with physical, social, and personal functioning, it is not an applicable tool for adult family members who are not employed. Furthermore, soldier occupational functioning is directly relevant to readiness, but family members' occupational functioning, when applicable, represents just a single aspect of family readiness. However, because of its broad focus on overall functioning and its applicability to a working population, we nonetheless selected the WRFIS for further consideration for assessing soldier readiness. This decision also aligned with recommendations from BH experts and providers who thought that functioning—for example, job performance, relationships with friends and family, and the ability to work in teams—was an important aspect in measuring readiness.

### Potential Metric Using Walter Reed Functional Impairment Scale Data

We developed an example of a potential outcome metric that could be computed using WRFIS data and assessed it using our metric criteria described in Chapter Two (Table 4.3). The denominator of this outcome metric would include soldiers who receive BH care in an Army MTF (i.e., direct care) with a WRFIS score at or above a threshold level of severity (e.g., indicating at least moderate functional impairment). The numerator would include soldiers who have a specified decrease in WRFIS score within six months. The exact threshold score to be included in this metric would need to be defined, along with the point decrease that would indicate clinically meaningful improvement in functioning. This example metric is similar to the "response-to-treatment" outcome metrics currently tracked by the Army, which evaluate whether symptoms improve for patients with particular diagnoses (i.e., PTSD, depression, or anxiety). These response-to-treatment metrics are modeled after an NQF-endorsed measure that assesses whether depression symptoms improved within six months (National Quality Forum, 2019a).

We applied the criteria in Table 2.1 to evaluate this example metric using WRFIS data (Table 4.2).

- *Importance.* The WRFIS targets four domains of functioning related to the demands of military duty. As noted in Chapter One, readiness is a top concern of the Army, and it has set a goal to achieve a nondeployable rate of 5 percent or less. The example metric addresses a high-priority area in which there is an opportunity to improve.

**Table 4.3**
**Example Readiness Metric Using Walter Reed Functional Impairment Scale Data**

**Metric numerator:** soldiers with a specified improvement in WRFIS score within six months

**Metric denominator:** soldiers in BH care with a threshold severity WRFIS score

| Evaluation Criteria | | | | | |
|---|---|---|---|---|---|
| Important | Feasible | Valid | Reliable | Sensitive to Change | Usable |
| Yes | Yes | 14-item WRFIS: Yes<br>6-item WRFIS: No data<br>Metric: Unable to determine | 14-item WRFIS: Yes<br>6-item WRFIS: No data<br>Metric: Unable to determine | No data | No data |

- *Feasibility.* The self-report data to support this example metric are retrievable without undue burden or cost since BHDP currently contains a shorter 8-item version of the WRFIS. The data can be collected from soldiers routinely while receiving BH care at an MTF. Data can be accessed by Army BH leadership and/or DHA.
- *Scientific acceptability.* The 14-item WRFIS appears to have some degree of *validity* based on the initial development work. The instrument has face validity, in that it was developed specifically to assess functioning in service members. The incorporation of multiple domains to assess a concept that is thought to involve different aspects of functioning provides support for content validity. There is also evidence of criterion validity in that it correlates with BH symptoms and social and occupational performance outcomes. The 14-item WRFIS has also shown high internal consistency *reliability* (Cronbach's $\alpha$ = 0.92) (Herrell et al., 2014). Further tests of its psychometric properties and those of the 6-item version are in progress. Currently there are no data to establish the example metric's *sensitivity to change.*
- *Usability.* Although the WRFIS is currently included in BHDP, we do not have current information about its level of use by providers. Its perceived utility to providers and the Army as a useful source of data to monitor soldier readiness is unknown. As noted earlier, the WRFIS is not applicable as a monitor of family readiness.

The lack of data about the WRFIS sensitivity to change and its usability are notable limitations to a WRFIS-based readiness metric. To consider using the WRFIS as a readiness metric, further analyses and pilot testing are needed. Further work has been done to evaluate the psychometrics of the 14-item and 6-item versions of the WRFIS and their comparison with the RAND VR-12. When these data are available, they will provide more information to assess the WRFIS's potential use. The 8-item version (which includes the items in the 6-item version) is currently part of BHDP and would have less burden of completion than the full 14-item version. Additionally, the BHDP database currently contains 8-item WRFIS data for a sample of soldiers who have received BH care. Given these factors, a plan to examine these data and pilot a potential metric is described in Box 4.1. Implementation of these pilot testing steps will also ensure that a WRFIS-based readiness metric adds value over the existing symptom-based outcome metrics.

## Evaluating eProfile as a Potential Source of Readiness Data

The current data system that records when soldiers are not ready to deploy is the eProfile system. A module within MODS, eProfile enables users to track soldiers who have a temporary or permanent medical condition that may make them medically unready for a deployment.

## Box 4.1 Plan for Pilot Testing a WRFIS-based Readiness Metric

### Step 1: Assess Current Level of Use of the WRFIS in Army BH Care

*Goal: to determine the level of provider implementation of the WRFIS and effort that will be needed to increase use of the instrument.*

- Using WRFIS data in BHDP, compute:
  - percentage of soldiers seen in Army BH care with at least one administration; at least two administrations
  - mean number of completed WRFIS administrations per patient, frequency distribution.
- Assess whether level of implementation varies by MTF. Consider conducting qualitative interviews with BH providers at MTFs that use the measure more frequently to assess clinical utility.

### Step 2: Conduct Descriptive Analyses of Existing WRFIS Data

*Goal: to evaluate psychometric properties of the WRFIS in soldiers receiving Army BH care and inform outcome metric specifications.*

- Using available WRFIS scores in BHDP, compute
  - mean, median total scores
  - interval consistency reliability (e.g., Cronbach's $\alpha$).
- Assess concurrent validity by evaluating how WRFIS scores relate to other key variables by computing correlations between a soldier's WRFIS score and:
  - symptom scores (e.g., PHQ-9 item, PTSD Checklist, Generalized Anxiety Disorder–7 item, Couples Symptom Inventory)
  - number of BH diagnoses (as an indicator of comorbidity).
- Assess predicative validity by evaluating how WRFIS scores (i.e., a soldier's last score) predict ability to deploy and separation
- Among soldiers with at least two administered the WRFIS, evaluate sensitivity to change and compute:
  - mean initial WRFIS score
  - mean last WRFIS score
  - mean WRFIS score change (i.e., last WRFIS score minus first score)
  - percentage of soldiers with specified decreases in WRFIS score 4–8 months after initial score.

---

**Box 4.1—Continued**

**Step 3: Define Detailed Metric Specifications**

*Goal: to develop detailed outcome metric specifications to increase the likelihood that the metric meets metric evaluation criteria (e.g., scientific acceptability).*

- Define population eligible for metric (denominator):
  - eligible BH diagnoses (e.g., PTSD, depression, anxiety)
  - eligible episode of care (e.g., beginning a new treatment episode vs. ongoing care)
  - type of BH visit and/or type of provider
  - minimum number and timing of WRFIS administrations (e.g., two required—initial administration plus at least one additional 4–8 months later)
  - minimum threshold WRFIS score for inclusion (e.g., score that indicates impaired functioning, such as ≥20 for the 14-item version).
- Define required improvement in WRFIS score that would indicate treatment response (numerator)
  - score-point decrease (or percent decrease) that would indicate clinically significant improvement in functioning.
- Compute metric scores

**Step 4: Pilot Test Metric**

*Goal: to assess whether the metric provides useful readiness-related information to monitor and improve BH care.*

- Given current rates of implementation, assess whether metric can be tested Army-wide or whether testing should be conducted with a few target MTFs (perhaps with higher rates of current WRFIS use).
- Compute metric scores and evaluate how metric scores relate to symptom-based metrics (e.g., PTSD, depression, anxiety symptom metrics assessing response to treatment and remission).

---

Army Regulation 40-501—Medical Services, Standards of Medical Fitness (2017) provides guidelines for when medical conditions warrant placing a soldier on a profile, and the U.S. Army Medical Command (MEDCOM) 2017 policy on standardizing profiles for BH conditions and recent updates to determining readiness and medical deployability (Secretary of the Army, 2018) provide additional instruction. Profiles can be either temporary or permanent, and they are assigned a level ranging from 1 to 4 depending on functional capacity. Permanent profile levels derive from PULHES scores (military medical grading system), where PULHES represent six organs or systems of the body (P = physical capacity or stamina; U = upper extremities; L = lower extremities; H = hearing and ears; E = eyes; and S = psychiatric). If all six organs or systems are level 1, the profile will be a 1 indicating that the individual "is considered to possess a high level of medical fitness" (Army Regulation 40-501—Medical Services, Standards of Medical Fitness, 2017). Any PULHES score of 2 translates to a physical profile of 2, meaning the "individual possess some medical condition of physical defect that may require some activity limitations" (Army Regulation 40-501—Medical Services, Standards of Medical Fitness, 2017). A designation of 3 on a PULHES factor, corresponding to a profile of 3, indicates that the service member has "one or more medical conditions of physical defects that may require significant limitations" and that "the individual should receive assignment commensurate with his or her physical capacity for military duty" (Army Regulation 40-501—Medical Services, Standards of Medical Fitness, 2017). Finally, a profile of 4, corresponding to one or more PULHES scores of 4, means "the individual has one or more medical conditions or physical defects of such severity that performance of military duty must be drastically limited" (Army Regulation 40-501—Medical Services, Standards of Medical Fitness, 2017). Therefore, permanent profiles take on such values as P3 (permanent, level 3). The level of the profile (1–4) does not automatically indicate whether the soldier is deployable, what his or her assignment restrictions are, or whether he or she needs to be referred for disability evaluation; the specific medical condition and the soldier's functional limitations determine their capabilities (Army Regulation 40-501—Medical Services, Standards of Medical Fitness, 2017). Temporary profiles do not derive from PULHES scores (U.S. Army, 2017). Instead, the reason for a temporary profile is now documented using a template, which contains extensive guidance for writing the profile and allows the provider to document the soldier's duty restrictions.

MEDCOM's 2017 BH eProfiling Standardization Policy memo states that a soldier's medical readiness for duty will be assessed during every clinical encounter. It defines the minimum assessment that must be done, including "the Soldier's mental status, risk of harm to self or others, symptom severity, prognosis for return to full duty, treatment needs, and risk of decompensation or further injury if the soldier participates in occupational activities" (U.S. Army, 2017, p. 3). It also describes the specific circumstances under which profiles should be issued related to BH conditions. This guidance is generally about when a temporary profile should be issued (e.g., when the soldier is at risk of harm to self or others, but duty restrictions will mitigate the risk), what profile to issue when a soldier is not expected to meet medical retention standards within a year of diagnosis, the profile requirements for a soldier on psychotropic medication, and determinations that define a soldier's ability to deploy.

In addition to this guidance, the policy memo contains two enclosures, one that provides examples of appropriate documentation of functional limitations and rationale, which providers are encouraged to include in profile comments, and a second that describes minimal profile guidance. The minimal profile guidance instructs providers when to place a soldier on a profile and when to reassess or renew the profile. For example, for several BH conditions, the soldier is to be placed on a 90-day profile and reassessed at the end of that period to determine if a permanent profile is warranted. For other conditions, the soldier is to remain on temporary profile until he or she is removed from at-risk case tracking.

### Interview Respondent Perspectives on eProfile

We asked BH experts what existing data could be used to support the development of a metric to assess readiness among those who have received BH care. Most ($n = 15$) indicated that being on a profile was an indicator of medical nonreadiness. Profiles were also viewed by some as a useful tool for communicating duty limitations to the soldier's commander.

However, BH experts and providers also indicated a number of concerns about using profile data to support a readiness metric. First, respondents reported a lack of consistency in how profiles are applied, which limits the utility of what profiles (or the lack of a profile) convey. One respondent suggested that the length of time a soldier is on a profile can be a readiness indicator, but since different diagnoses have different recovery trajectories, profile duration alone may not indicate anything about readiness. Finally, one respondent reported that the Army developed metrics to explore whether providers were correctly applying profiles to all soldiers who should have been on them, based on information available in MODS and the MHS Data Repository (e.g., admitted to inpatient facility for a limiting condition or received deployment-limiting medication). One study found some evidence of soldiers who should have been on profile but were not (Curley and Warner, 2017). In the next chapter, we discuss eProfile in more detail and present recommendations from respondents about ways to improve how profiles are applied.

### Potential Metric Using eProfile Data

Since the presence of a BH profile indicates that a soldier is not ready, coming off a profile upon the completion of BH care—and not going back on a BH profile within a set period of time—may suggest that the soldier is now ready and that, at least in part, treatment provided while on the profile was effective. Based on this assumption, we developed an example of a potential metric using profile data and assessed it using our metric criteria described in Chapter Two (Table 4.4). In this example metric, the denominator includes soldiers in BH care who have been placed on a BH profile, and the numerator includes those soldiers who are *not* on a BH profile six months later.

- *Importance.* The example metric targets functioning and readiness-related demands of military duty. As noted earlier, levels of readiness are top priority, and the Army has set a target benchmark. The metric measures a high-priority area in which there is an opportunity to improve.

**Table 4.4**
**Example Readiness Metric Using eProfile Data**

**Metric Numerator:** soldiers who are not on a BH profile in six months

**Metric Denominator:** soldiers in BH care who are placed on a BH profile

| Evaluation Criteria | | | | | |
|---|---|---|---|---|---|
| **Important** | **Feasible** | **Valid** | **Reliable** | **Sensitive to Change** | **Usable** |
| Yes | Unable to determine | Profile data: Unable to determine | Profile data: Unable to determine | No data | No data |
| | | Metric: Unable to determine | Metric: Unable to determine | | |

- *Feasibility.* The feasibility of using data from eProfile to construct a readiness metric is not known. Our interviews with BH experts did not reveal complete details about the content of eProfile data, and we did not have direct access to the data elements/variables that are currently available; therefore, our information about the specific data elements is somewhat incomplete.[2] Based on input from interview respondents' experience with the data, there appears to be some difficulties associated with accessing coded data from BH profiles. (Free text would not be suitable for this purpose.) In the absence of evaluating this information, we are unable to determine the feasibility of using eProfile data for this example metric. There were some promising aspects of feasibility. Specifically, policy guidance indicates that a soldier's readiness for duty should be assessed during every clinical encounter, suggesting that profiles should be updated as necessary to reflect current levels of readiness. This process is already integrated into the practices of Army providers. Further, Army BH leadership have access to eProfile data.
- *Scientific acceptability.* Profile data have face *validity*, in that profiling guidance and eProfile were designed specifically to document soldier readiness (i.e., by indicating lack of readiness). There is some indication that profiles have predictive validity, as soldiers with BH waivers to deploy (after being determined to not be medically ready) have been more likely than those without waivers to be medically evacuated from theater (Cronrath et al., 2017). This suggests that being on a profile measures lack of readiness. However, questions were raised about the *reliability* of profile data. Interviewed providers described inconsistency in the application of profiles, and an initiative to measure the application of BH profiles

---

[2]   We had access to a data dictionary intended to be used by external consumers of eProfile data, and it included variables about a soldier and their unit, characteristics of the symptom(s), date the condition started and ended, whether the condition is temporary or permanent, severity of the condition (if temporary), PULHES score, and functional and duty limitations. It is not clear how representative these variables are with respect to the universe of information available in eProfile.

revealed some underuse of profiles, which was consistent with what we learned during interviews. Instruments or data sources that are not reliable typically are not considered valid. Given this, we note that we are unable to determine the validity and reliability of profile data and this example metric. There are no data about eProfile data *sensitivity to change*.

- *Usability.* Although not all providers viewed profile data as a way to measure readiness, most did, and, therefore, we believe a metric created from eProfile data could be seen as meaningful and informative for providers. However, its usability as a metric is unknown.

Given the issues noted above, it is unclear whether eProfile data could be used to support a readiness metric. In any event, some improvements would have to be made to reduce some of eProfile's current shortcomings. Respondents expressed that profile guidance should be enhanced to more clearly identify when providers should write a profile, providers should be formally trained in when and how to write profiles, and the Army should monitor the application of profiles. As noted earlier, B-REDI is a decision support tool designed to help providers determine whether to write a profile for a soldier for a BH condition. The effectiveness of the B-REDI program is currently being evaluated. An assessment of B-REDI training provided at five sites in fall 2018 indicated high end-user satisfaction with training and a significant improvement in provider knowledge, confidence, and decisionmaking regarding applying profile policy posttraining (Curley, 2019). Respondents also indicated that profiles and diagnoses are not entered into the same system; eProfile captures profiles, and related diagnoses are entered into the Armed Forces Health Longitudinal Technology Application. If the two systems were integrated, providers would not have to switch between systems to enter data that are inherently related. The reader should note that integrating these systems may not be feasible due to confidentiality requirements. Finally, because profiles relate directly to soldier readiness, metrics drawn from eProfile data would not be applicable to family readiness.

## Results of the Search to Identify Potential Instruments to Measure Readiness

As described in Chapter Two, our search of the literature targeted the identification of instruments used to assess readiness in military service members and their families. The search resulted in 14 articles that met final inclusion criteria and contained 50 instruments used in military populations that addressed functioning or readiness. The extracted data about these instruments were evaluated to explore the feasibility and application for soldiers and adult family members who received BH care. To remain in consideration, an instrument needed to be self-report, contain no more than 30 items, and assess readiness/functioning. Few instruments met the standard of assess-

**Table 4.5**
**Candidate Instruments from the Instrument Search That Were Excluded**

| Instrument | Description | Final Exclusion Criterion |
|---|---|---|
| CD-RISC-25: Connor-Davidson Resilience Scale | Resilience metric with factors related to competence, tolerance of negative affect, change and relationships, control, and spiritual influences | Proprietary tool |
| DRS-15: Dispositional Resilience Scale | Hardiness metric with subscales for commitment, control, and challenge | Proprietary tool |

ing the broader concept of readiness/functioning. (See Appendix E for a list of instruments considered and the reasons for their exclusion.) Given the emphasis on resilience as a readiness factor related to the ability to adapt to stressors and meet changing demands in both soldiers and adult family members (Chairman of the Joint Chiefs of Staff Instruction 3405.01, 2011; Meadows et al., 2016), we identified two instruments that measured resilience, described in Table 4.5: the Connor-Davidson Resilience Scale (CD-RISC; CDRISC, undated; Connor and Davidson, 2003) and the Dispositional Resilience Scale (DRS; Bartone, 2008; Bartone, 2007). However, both instruments are proprietary tools. Therefore, none of the instruments in the literature that had been used with military populations or their families met final inclusion criteria for further consideration.

## Results of Supplemental Search

The complete list resulting from our supplemental search for recommended instruments to measure functioning can be found in Appendix F. Three instruments were within our 30-item limit and have been used with various populations (Table 4.6). These include two instruments from the Patient-Reported Outcomes Measurement Information System (PROMIS) and the World Health Organization Disability Assessment Schedule (WHODAS) 2.0 (Cella et al., 2010; Hays et al., 2009; World Health Organization, 2010). PROMIS Global Health and PROMIS-29 are from the PROMIS item banks of outcome measures for commonly studied patient-reported outcomes. Both instruments incorporate domains of physical and mental health, fatigue, pain, and social roles. PROMIS-29 also includes a domain assessing sleep disturbance. WHODAS 2.0 collects self-report responses about difficulty functioning (in terms of cognition, mobility, self-care, getting along, life activities, and participation) due to health conditions.

All three instruments are meant to assess health status and disability in community-dwelling adults in both clinical and population settings. The physical domains of these instruments include items addressing activities of daily living, such as the ability to

**Table 4.6**
**Candidate Instruments from Supplemental Search That Were Excluded**

| Instrument | Description | Source | Final Exclusion Criterion |
|---|---|---|---|
| PROMIS Global Health | Patient self-report of general health, physical health, mental health, social/work, fatigue, and pain | Subject-matter expert recommendation | Focus on limitations due to health conditions |
| PROMIS-29 Profile | Collection of four-item short forms assessing physical functioning, anxiety, depression, fatigue, pain, sleep disturbance, and social roles | Subject-matter expert recommendation | Focus on limitations due to health conditions |
| WHODAS 2.0 | Patient self-report of physical, emotional, and social/ occupational functioning | International Consortium for Health Outcomes Measurement and Kennedy Forum | Focus on limitations due to health conditions |

walk and bathe oneself, and instrumental activities of daily living, such as the ability to run errands or buy groceries. Because the populations of interest for this study (soldiers and families) are comprised of younger adults, predominantly physically able and functioning in a unique military environment that is distinct from that of civilians, we judged the PROMIS and WHODAS tools to not be sufficiently relevant for assessing functioning relative to readiness. Therefore, none of the instruments identified from the supplemental search met final inclusion criteria for further consideration.

## Summary

In this chapter, we reviewed and evaluated the possibility of using an existing data source to construct a readiness metric. We suggested an example outcome metric constructed using WRFIS data contained in BHDP, which would focus on improvement in functioning, and an example metric making use of profile or duty limitation data. However, a WRFIS-based metric would require continued study of the WRFIS's psychometric properties and existing WFRIS data to determine its usefulness for tracking readiness. Data from eProfile are currently used to identify soldiers who are not ready and could potentially be used to construct a new readiness metric. However, improvements in the reliable application of BH profiles and accessibility of coded eProfile data would be needed prior to the use of eProfile data for this purpose. While both sources include data related to soldier readiness, neither data source is designed to support a readiness metric for adult family members.

This chapter also presented the results of our targeted search of the literature, which focused on existing instruments that could support a readiness metric for either service members or adult family members. During our full text review, only two instruments (CD-RISC and DRS) met the initial criteria for being self-report, containing no more than 30 items, and assessing readiness or functioning. However, both are proprietary tools and were therefore screened out as well. We also conducted a supplemental search for instruments that measure functioning (more generally, not necessarily within a military population) that were recommended in core sets of BH outcome instruments and other metrics suggested by BH experts. Using the same criteria that we applied to the instruments from the search of the literature, we identified three instruments: PROMIS Global Health, PROMIS-29, and WHODAS 2.0. We concluded that none of the three was useful to assess readiness of soldiers and their families. Because the populations of interest for this study (soldiers and adult family members) are comprised of younger adults, who are predominantly physically able and functioning in a unique military environment that is distinct from that of civilians, we judged the PROMIS and WHODAS instruments to not be sufficiently relevant for assessing functioning relative to readiness.

# CHAPTER FIVE

# Improving Readiness Assessment

Although the primary objective of this project was to identify metrics to assess readiness among soldiers and adult family members who receive BH care, our interviews offered an opportunity to document stakeholder perspectives on how readiness assessment could be improved. In this chapter, we describe findings from interviews with both BH experts and providers on the way to improve readiness assessment.

## Behavioral Health Expert and Provider Views on Improving Readiness Assessment

Following the discussion of indicators of readiness and ways to assess and measure it, we asked BH experts ($N = 18$) and BH providers ($N = 24$) what improvements could be made to how readiness is currently assessed for soldiers who receive BH care. Respondents had a number of suggestions that can be categorized into seven themes:

- improving the functioning and utility of measures and data systems
- improving communication between medical providers and the soldier's operational command
- improving provider consistency in following military policy or guidelines
- improving policies or guidelines
- increasing resources for providers
- improving prevention or increasing treatment for soldiers
- providing more support to families.

Within each of these themes, there was a small number of topics mentioned by several respondents and a wide variety of other suggestions that were mentioned by only one or two. In this section, we report on the specific topics mentioned by relatively larger numbers of respondents, but topics mentioned by just one or two are discussed at a higher level (i.e., groups of topics that form a subtheme within a theme), highlighting only a subset of the more specific suggestions for improvement.

**Utility of Data Systems**

The area mentioned most frequently for improvement was the functioning and utility of measures and data systems. Nearly all BH experts and almost 80 percent of BH providers had suggestions for improving measures and data systems for assessing readiness (BH experts, $n$ = 17; BH providers, $n$ = 19). The topics centered on specific data systems, such as BHDP and eProfile (BH experts, $n$ = 12; BH providers, $n$ = 16) and expanding the information available for making a readiness determination (BH experts, $n$ = 16; BH providers, $n$ = 10). Improvements to BHDP included expanding the BHDP portal (BH experts, $n$ = 9; BH providers, $n$ = 14), such as adding contact information for commanders and improving the performance of the system (e.g., reported to run slowly and not update graphs with screening tool data). Other suggestions related to expanding the information in BHDP about the soldier's MOS, identifying soldiers who might be at risk or need BH care based on prior history, and integrating BHDP and eProfile so that providers did not have to switch between systems during a patient encounter.

The second way respondents thought measures and data systems could be improved was by making more information available to the provider for making a readiness determination. The most common response in this area was about information on family members (BH experts, $n$ = 7; BH providers, $n$ = 16), including whether they are ready for the soldier to deploy, the level of support they required, and whether they are satisfied with military life. Knowing whether the family feels ready for the soldier to deploy supports an earlier interview finding about what readiness means for family members; many respondents indicated that if the adult family member cannot function independently (without the soldier), that would be an indicator that the adult family member is not ready. Another improvement that was suggested related to family readiness was the development of a profile system for adult family members. There were also a number of responses about additional data on soldiers that could improve the way readiness is assessed. For example, half of all BH experts recommended improving BH data collection, such as tracking the number of BH visits and including information about soldiers who had BH issues during a prior deployment or were medically evacuated for BH reasons (BH experts, $n$ = 9; BH providers, $n$ = 2). Other suggestions included collecting information on functioning (e.g., job performance) (BH experts, $n$ = 5; BH providers, $n$ = 2), financial stability (BH experts, $n$ = 2; BH providers, $n$ = 2), infractions and administrative actions (BH experts, $n$ = 2; BH providers, $n$ = 2), and allowing the provider access to complete data for a full medical review when making a readiness determination (BH experts, $n$ = 3; BH providers, $n$ = 3) (e.g., to identify potential red flags, such as past psychiatric hospitalizations). Finally, a number of respondents recommended collecting self-reports on whether the soldier feels ready to deploy (BH experts, $n$ = 5; BH providers, $n$ = 2) and whether the soldier wants to stay in the military (BH experts, $n$ = 3; BH providers, $n$ = 2).

## Communication with Commanders

The next most-discussed area for improving the way readiness is assessed pertained to the relationship between medical providers and the soldier's operational command. More than one-third of BH experts and BH providers (BH experts, $n = 7$; BH providers, $n = 9$) mentioned a possible improvement in this area, either related to communication between the medical providers and operational command (BH experts, $n = 3$; BH providers, $n = 8$) or more generally about increased engagement between the two (BH experts, $n = 4$; BH providers, $n = 4$). BH experts and BH providers seemed to agree that improved communication (in general) between the medical provider and operational commander would help with assessing readiness (BH experts, $n = 2$; BH providers, $n = 4$). Other suggestions related to communication mentioned by smaller numbers of respondents included earlier communication regarding where the soldier would be deploying (including the command's requirements for that location) and earlier communication regarding readiness concerns to avoid a situation where the soldier feels unable to deploy days before his or her assignment begins. Respondents also had some suggestions about how BH providers could engage the operational command. For example, respondents suggested it would be helpful if commanders had increased awareness about the potential value of BH care in supporting soldier readiness. Respondents mentioned that a reduced use of stigmatizing language related to BH care, in addition to better communication and mutual understanding of BH care, could help minimize differences in perspectives regarding a soldier's readiness.

## Military Policy and Guidelines

About 40 percent of BH experts and 20 percent of BH providers thought that another area for improvement was the consistency with which providers followed military policy or guidelines (BH experts, $n = 7$; BH providers, $n = 5$). Specifically, respondents reported variation in how providers applied profile standards (BH experts, $n = 4$; BH providers, $n = 1$), and they thought providers could benefit from additional education on the functional expectations for the soldier in the context of the military mission (BH experts, $n = 5$; BH providers, $n = 4$).

Half of BH providers recommended improvements in policy (BH experts, $n = 2$; BH providers, $n = 12$), including both operational guidelines (BH experts, $n = 2$; BH providers, $n = 8$) and medical guidelines (BH providers, $n = 5$). Improved screening at the time of enlistment was the policy-related suggestion mentioned by the largest number of respondents (BH experts, $n = 1$; BH providers, $n = 6$). Operational guidelines that respondents thought should be improved included harmonizing deployment standards (e.g., creating a common standard for all geographic locations) and reducing the wait time between when a soldier is deemed not ready and when they are removed from the military (if appropriate). One operational guideline for families that a respondent mentioned improving was making enrollment in the Exceptional Family Member Program (a program to support families with unique needs) provider driven rather than soldier driven. This would allow providers the ability to enroll family members rather than relying on the soldier to initiate this process. A small number of respondents had other policy-related suggestions, such as allowing a review of BH care prior to reenlistment and harmonizing deployment policies with respect to medication treatment (e.g., across geographic commands). Another example that one interviewee mentioned was changing the timeline for substance use and deployment standards. Currently, Army policy states that soldiers who enroll in SUDCC cannot deploy for 12 months (USCENTCOM MOD 13, Tab A; U.S. Central Command, 2017); this policy can be a challenge for providers because severity of illness and response to treatment varies by soldier.

### Resources and Support Services

The final three themes had a smaller number of overall responses, predominantly from BH providers. For example, one-fifth of BH providers thought additional resources should be made available for providers (BH experts, $n = 1$; BH providers, $n = 6$), such as more staff, computers, and the time and ability to do more psychological testing. A similar number of BH providers recommended increased prevention or treatment for soldiers (BH experts, $n = 1$; BH providers, $n = 5$). The most common suggestion within this theme was increased access to care for soldiers and family members (BH experts, $n = 1$; BH providers, $n = 4$), but other responses were about more prevention through psychoeducation for soldiers and getting soldiers who are identified as in need of care into treatment.

Although this question focused on improving readiness assessment for soldiers, the last theme was about providing more support to families (BH experts, $n = 1$; BH providers, $n = 3$). BH experts and BH providers both thought families would benefit from additional education about what to expect regarding soldier deployment and the supportive resources available to them (BH experts, $n = 1$; BH providers, $n = 3$). Another suggestion in this area was to have families complete or be assessed by a readiness checklist prior to the soldier's deployment to assess the level of family readiness and, if needed, to target appropriate resources for the family. This last topic within this theme, although mentioned by a small number of respondents, relates to suggested improvements discussed earlier regarding additional data collection to supplement making a readiness determination, especially the recommendation to ask family members if they are ready for their soldier to deploy.

### Summary

When asked about possible improvements to how readiness is assessed, BH experts and providers offered a wide range of ideas. The most common responses were to expand the information available in BHDP or improve the portal's utility and to increase the amount of information collected on family members. One suggested way to expand or improve BHDP was to add contact information for commanders, something that would support other recommendations to expand communication between the BH provider and the operational command. Other suggestions included improving the system's technical performance, collecting more information about the soldier's MOS (which would provide clarity on job requirements), and integrating BHDP with eProfile. There were other recommendations for additional data collection, such as the number of BH visits and whether the soldier experienced BH problems during a prior deployment or was medically evacuated for BH reasons. Along with expanding BHDP, these recommendations fall under a larger category of making more information available to support readiness determinations.

Finally, because there is not currently a way to measure family readiness, the suggestion to gather more information from families about factors that affect their readiness would help fill that gap. The most commonly suggested data concerned whether family members are satisfied with military life and whether they are ready for the soldier to deploy, but some respondents thought that a family profile should be created and that families should complete or be assessed on a checklist prior to the soldier's deployment to identify the need for resources to ensure readiness.

# CHAPTER SIX

# Summary and Recommendations

In this chapter, we highlight the strengths and limitations of our project methods, highlight our main findings, and provide recommendations for how the Army can continue to improve outcomes for soldiers who receive BH care.

We employed several methods to help the Army identify potential approaches to measuring readiness for soldiers and adult family members who received BH care, which would, in turn, help assess the effectiveness of BH care in supporting readiness in this population. First, we defined the criteria by which we would evaluate a potential readiness metric. Then, we interviewed BH experts and providers on a range of topics, including indicators of readiness for both soldiers and adult family members, information used to make a readiness determination, how providers interact with commanders in assessing readiness, readiness metrics that could be derived from existing data, and ways to improve readiness assessment. We also conducted an independent search for existing data that could potentially support a readiness metric, searched the literature for instruments that have been used to assess the readiness of soldiers or adult family members, and conducted a supplemental search for instruments that measure functioning in the general population. We used all these sources of information to narrow down to two potential existing data sources that could support a soldier readiness metric and applied a set of criteria to evaluate example metrics to determine whether they could be recommended for implementation.

## Strengths and Limitations

There are several strengths associated with the methods we employed. With the interviews of BH experts and BH providers, we were able to discern and consider the input of stakeholders on various facets of readiness, its assessment, and potential improvements. When considering potential outcome metrics, we applied rigorous criteria to evaluate them based on their importance, feasibility, scientific acceptability, and usability. This is important given the challenges and costs of implementing any outcome metric and the risks associated with using metrics that are not psychometrically sound and perceived as usable.

There are also some limitations that should be noted. First, the project focused only on the readiness of soldiers and adult family members. This is a limitation in that the readiness of children and adolescents is a key part of overall family readiness. Second, because this project was sponsored by the Army, we focused on Army readiness policies and practices and interviewed Army BH experts and providers; therefore, our findings may not be applicable across other service branches. Third, our findings are based on a limited number of interviews, 18 BH experts and 24 BH providers, some of whom had little or no experience working with adult family members. We had hoped to interview commanders to understand the operational perspective on readiness, but we were unable to arrange those interviews within the project timeline. Further, perspectives of soldiers and adult family members would have also been useful. Finally, because readiness represents a unique type of functioning compared with that in the nonmilitary community, we applied strict criteria to our instrument search, such as requiring readiness to be mentioned in the project. Therefore, we may have missed some sources, particularly instruments used with adults outside of the military that could have warranted consideration. We did aim to overcome this limitation by conducting a supplemental search, which in the end produced results that were less applicable to a young, generally healthy military population.

## Findings

### Stakeholders Reported That Psychiatric Symptoms, Diagnoses, Treatment, and Impaired Functioning Are Important Indicators of Lack of Readiness for Soldiers and Adult Family Members

When asked about conceptual indicators of readiness, BH experts and BH providers cited psychiatric symptoms or diagnoses and related treatment as indicators of not being ready for both soldiers and adult family members. These included psychiatric symptoms related to risk (e.g., suicidal ideation) and specific BH diagnoses (e.g., PTSD, depression, SUD) with high symptom severity, need for intensive psychiatric treatment, or treatment with certain psychotropic medications. These responses reflected the Army's current policies regarding BH conditions and their potential negative impact on readiness. For soldiers and family members receiving care from an MTF, the Army uses BHDP to collect data on symptoms for several BH conditions (e.g., PTSD, depression, anxiety), as well as other BH-related symptoms (e.g., insomnia, couple satisfaction, general distress). Findings from stakeholder interviews highlight the importance of the Army's ongoing symptom monitoring as a key component of monitoring readiness for soldiers and adult family members.

However, the input regarding conceptual indicators of readiness also highlighted the significant role of multiple aspects of functioning, including occupational functioning (particularly for soldiers), social functioning, and general functioning (particularly for family members) related to readiness. Assessment of different aspects of functioning has been a focus of several published outcome metrics. For example, many of the NQF-endorsed outcome metrics focus on functioning in selected circumstances or populations, such as metrics to assess functioning after total knee replacement surgery, in those with rheumatoid arthritis, or for those in inpatient rehabilitation (National Quality Forum, 2019b). Other instruments used in general populations focus on more overall functioning, but with a focus on the impact of or disability related to physical and/or mental illness, such as the WHODAS 2.0 described earlier in this report. The Centers for Medicare and Medicaid Services is currently partnering with clinicians and professional societies to develop new meaningful quality measures, including outcome metrics. One metric in the conceptual stage, with an estimated date of completion of fall 2021, is improvement or maintenance of functioning for all patients seen for mental health and substance use care. This metric is being developed in collaboration with the American Psychiatric Association (Center for Clinical Standards and Quality, 2019).

In a separate effort, the American Psychological Association has developed a Mental and Behavioral Health Registry (MBHR) to collect clinical data about the health status of patients and to facilitate participation in value-based programs, such as the Centers for Medicare and Medicaid Services' Merit-Based Incentive Payment System (Wright et al., 2019). Assessment of functioning is also a priority for inclusion in the MBHR. To address the gap of measures of functioning for BH care, the American Psychological Association is incorporating patient-reported measures on three domains of functional impairment: pain, sleep, and social functioning in MBHR as non–Merit-Based Incentive Payment System measures (American Psychological Association, 2019).[1] The various efforts described here highlight the importance of assessing functioning but also indicate the ongoing challenges of measuring a construct that is multidimensional and complex and the absence of established outcome metrics that assess functioning in patients who receive BH care. In the case of the Army, the challenge of identifying a metric of functioning is further complicated by the unique demands the military places on soldiers and their adult family members.

**No Existing Data Source or Patient Self-Report Instrument Met Criteria for Army-Wide Implementation of a Readiness Metric for Soldiers, but One Instrument Is Promising**

Implementation of an outcome metric can be challenging for an organization and involves an investment in resources to support those efforts. Collecting new data and developing a new metric using those data to monitor readiness would be a worthwhile effort if the instrument used and its associated outcome metric was scientifically tested and accepted (as valid, reliable, and sensitive to change) for its intended pur-

---

[1]  The MBHR measure focused on social functioning is referenced in Appendix F.

pose. Therefore, we used rigorous criteria to evaluate whether any existing data sources would support a readiness metric for soldiers and/or adult family members.

We identified 15 existing data sources covering duty limitations (profiles), medical encounters, screeners and assessments, and other data related to health and readiness. We screened the 15 sources based on the population included in the data (soldiers, family members, active or reserve components), the frequency of data collection, applicability of the data to address readiness, and accessibility of the data to DHA leadership. Based on these criteria, we narrowed down the 15 existing data sources to 2 that could potentially support a readiness metric: the WRFIS contained within BHDP and profile data in eProfile.

We provided an example of how WRFIS data might be used to calculate a metric that assesses the percentage of soldiers receiving BH care with a threshold WRFIS severity score (i.e., indicating impairment in functioning) who have a meaningful improvement in the score within six months. The WRFIS (available in an original and short form) assesses important components of soldier readiness, is feasible to use, and appears valid and reliable (based on psychometric properties of the original form). Unfortunately, there are no data about either form of the instrument regarding sensitivity to change (i.e., scores improve over time in response to effective treatment), its usability as a clinical tool for providers to inform care for individual patients, and its applicability to assessing readiness. Therefore, before it could be implemented across the Army (or DoD-wide), some additional work is needed before the WRFIS could be used to assess readiness. Continuing the current work on assessing the psychometric properties of both the original and short version of the WRFIS will be valuable. Once these parameters are established, a pilot would be a useful way to test whether the WRFIS could support a readiness metric. Details of what this pilot could entail are summarized in Chapter Three. The results of the preliminary work on instrument psychometrics could inform the creation of a potential outcome metric to track soldier readiness using WRFIS data that could then be pilot tested.

An example of how profile data might be used to track soldier readiness would be the percentage of soldiers in BH care on a BH profile who are not on a BH profile six months later. However, like WRFIS data, any metric involving profiles is not yet ready for implementation. Our interviews with stakeholders and other existing research have identified some inconsistencies in how profiles are applied, leading to concerns about the reliability and validity of these data. For example, a recent review found that some soldiers who should have been on a profile, based on policy guidance, were not on a profile (Curley and Warner, 2017). Additional provider training to achieve greater consistency in how providers apply profiles would first need to be addressed.

## No Existing Data Source or Patient Self-Report Instrument Met Criteria for Army-Wide Implementation of a Readiness Metric for Adult Family Members

Neither the WRFIS nor profile data (both suggested as having potential for creating a readiness metric for soldiers) would support a readiness metric for adult family members. A recent qualitative analysis of indicators of family readiness identified 16 domains of functioning, including adult physical and mental health, social support, couple functioning, parenting/children's/family functioning, deployment-related experiences, finances and spouse employment, military life experiences, and accessibility of military services. Key findings highlighted the significance to family readiness of social support, marital quality and stability, and comprehensive programs to support all family members (Hawkins et al., 2018). The demands of military readiness on families are unique compared with the functional demands of civilian populations. Instruments to measure functioning in general populations tend to focus on limitations related to physical and mental health problems, including the impact on activities of daily living and instrumental activities of daily living, making them less relevant to military adult family members, who are likely to be young and in generally good health. In addition, the development of instruments to measure overall functioning, including in the context of BH care, is still evolving. Therefore, we found no existing self-report instrument to recommend for Army-wide implementation to monitor family readiness at this time.

## Behavioral Health Providers Reported Some Variability in Assessing Readiness, but Behavioral Health Experts and Providers Offered Suggestions for Improving Readiness Assessment

BH providers reported using similar information to assess readiness and when deciding whether to place a soldier on a profile, including occupational functioning, policy guidance, and collateral information, such as consulting with the soldier's command and, to a lesser extent, friends and family. The most common information used to assess readiness, however, was patient self-report measures and clinical interviews, which providers use to assess the patient's clinical presentation, determine diagnoses, and inform the treatment plan. Psychiatric symptoms and diagnoses, including risk and safety issues, are what the largest number of providers said they rely on for making a profile decision. Providers also mentioned that they consider current and past BH treatment, as documented in the medical record, when assessing readiness and making a profile decision. We asked BH providers if their view of soldier readiness ever differed from that of commanders. Most reported that differences in the roles and priorities of providers and commanders and differences in the way the soldier presents depending upon the setting do often result in different perspectives between the provider and commander.

When asked whether a soldier's specific duties inform the readiness decision and what influences whether a soldier is placed on a temporary or permanent profile, responses were more varied. The majority of providers responded that they rely on the soldier's MOS to determine specific duties, but some noted that MOS is too general to convey what the soldier must be able to do and instead rely on information from the command. Some providers felt that a soldier's specific duties are not relevant to assessing whether a soldier can deploy. Providers reported using a variety of information to determine whether to apply a permanent or temporary profile. Some generally use a temporary profile, especially during treatment, if there are concerns about how the soldier will perform during field training or because they could not or did not feel comfortable independently writing a permanent profile. On the other hand, some providers reported using permanent profiles if the soldier did not improve after being on a temporary profile, if they needed to be evaluated for disability, or if they were diagnosed with a chronic condition.

BH experts and BH providers had many suggestions for ways to improve the way readiness is assessed. Despite the variety of responses, two specific ideas stood out as having the most support, and many of the other ideas can be tied to these. The first is that BHDP should be improved for better performance technically and expanded to additional measures. There were also many other suggestions about gathering additional information about the soldier from other sources that is not currently included in or linked to BHDP but could be added to enhance the information that providers have when assessing readiness. The second idea mentioned by a large number of respondents was that more information should be collected about family members, including whether they are ready for their soldier to deploy. Other providers mentioned applying a checklist for the family (perhaps a self-evaluation or applied by a family support program) prior to deployment and developing a family profile system. All of these improvements would help to target needed family support services and fill a gap that exists today, which is that there is currently no means to measure family readiness.

## Recommendations

### Recommendation 1. Conduct a Pilot Evaluation of a WRFIS-Based Soldier Readiness Metric

The review of existing data sources revealed the inclusion of the 8-item WRFIS (which includes the items in the 6-item version) in BHDP. The original WRFIS was developed specifically to assess soldier functioning and assesses four domains including physical, occupational, personal, and social. We found the WRFIS to be a viable option for further work to develop a readiness metric. The WRFIS's specificity to soldier readiness and feasibility of use (e.g., brief length, currently available in BHDP, accessible to providers) are notable strengths. Further, we did not identify an alternative instrument suitable for soldiers and with adequate psychometric properties. Studies of the longer, 14-item WRFIS have indicated adequate validity and reliability of the instrument. Additional studies of the instrument and its short (6-item) version are currently in progress. We do not have current information about its level of use by providers. We recommend that the Army systematically test the use of the WRFIS as described in Chapter Three. Further testing would allow an assessment of the distribution of WRFIS scores, average change over time during BH care, and correlation with other symptoms scores. These analyses would guide the development of a potential metric to monitor soldier readiness that could be pilot tested in a defined population of those who receive Army BH care. These additional analyses would indicate the degree to which a WRFIS-based readiness metric is valid and sensitive to change. An approach for risk adjustment that takes into account differences in severity at treatment initiation would also need to be considered.

### Recommendation 2. Increase Standardization in Applying Profiles and Continue B-REDI Training

Profiles are used to communicate that a soldier has a medical condition that limits his or her ability to perform job-related duties. Therefore, profile data could be used to develop a metric that assesses and tracks soldier readiness. However, we learned during interviews that there are issues with the way profiles are applied. An Army assessment of whether BH profiles were being applied correctly determined that some soldiers who should have been on profiles were not (Curley and Warner, 2017). We recommend that before the Army considers using profile data to develop a readiness metric, steps should be taken to ensure that profiles are applied consistently across providers. Providers should receive additional training on when and how to place a soldier on a profile and continue provider decision support efforts. The B-REDI tool and associated training are an excellent example of the Army's efforts to standardize the application of profiles, and this effort should be continued.

## Directions for Future Research

The analyses presented in this report provide results that can guide the Army in improving outcomes for soldiers who receive BH care. These analyses also raised several questions that could be addressed in future research, including the following:

- *Conduct further development of the WRFIS.* We provide several next steps to evaluate the psychometrics properties of the WRFIS, along with a detailed plan to define a soldier readiness metric using WRFIS data. Additional research is needed to evaluate the WRFIS (particularly the short six-item version), including ensuring its psychometric properties are adequate, evaluating its clinical utility within a measurement-based care framework, and demonstrating that the instrument is sensitive to change.

- *Develop an instrument to assess readiness for adult family members.* Drawing on multiple data sources, including stakeholder interview and instrument search, this report highlights that the readiness of adult family members is a multidimensional construct. While readiness overlaps with functioning as typically conceived in civilians, there are unique aspects of the military family population and experience that warrant a readiness instrument specific to this population.
- *Assess the utility of profile data.* Profiles are a core strategy for communicating soldier readiness status to commanders. Yet there is limited information about the reliability and validity of profiles. Future research should evaluate the effectiveness of strategies to increase the reliability of applying profiles, such as B-REDI training. In addition, further evaluation of the validity of profiles is needed, such as examining how the presence or history of a profile predicts soldier service and BH outcomes. Further information is also needed on how effective BH care can affect whether a soldier remains on a profile (e.g., sensitivity to change).
- *Identify an approach to measuring the readiness of service members across service branches.* As noted in our limitations, we focused on identifying a potential readiness metric for soldiers, leading to a focus on Army providers, subject-matter experts, policies, and data systems. Administration of health care across service branches will be conducted by DHA, which has led to increased efforts to harmonize policies and oversight across the service branches. Additional research is needed to identify the commonalities and differences in definitions, policies, and practices related to medical readiness. This would support identifying potential metrics to assess service member readiness for service members who receive BH care through the MHS.
- *Capture other stakeholder perspectives to ensure outcome metrics in BH care assess important aspects of readiness.* Readiness is a multidimensional concept, and readiness outcome metrics within BH care should, if possible, assess aspects of readiness that are important across a variety of stakeholders. Conducting qualitative interviews with commanders and those who receive BH care (e.g., soldier, adult family members) would help to ensure that these metrics capture important aspects of readiness.

# Readiness Policies

## Table A.1
## Ready Soldiers and Families: Readiness Policies as of May 24, 2019

| Document Title | Publication Date or Effective Date | Description |
|---|---|---|
| Army Directive 2019-12 Policy for Voluntary Alcohol-Related Behavioral Healthcare | March 25, 2019 | Directive that describes "treating Soldiers who are voluntarily seeking alcohol-related behavioral healthcare. By distinguishing voluntary behavioral healthcare from mandatory enrolled substance abuse treatment, the Army will encourage Soldiers to seek help earlier and will improve readiness by decreasing unnecessary enrollment and deployment limitations." |
| Office of the Surgeon General (OTSG)/MEDCOM Policy Memo 19-010 Department of the Army Form 3822, Mental Status Evaluation | February 8, 2019 (expiration: February 8, 2021) | Policy memo to "provide guidance for behavioral healthcare providers and Military Treatment Facility (MTF) commanders on the use of the Department of the Army (DA) Form 3822 when conducting behavioral health (BH) evaluations." |
| OTSG/MEDCOM Policy Memo 19-001 Behavioral Health Evaluations for Administrative Separations of Active Duty Enlisted Soldiers under AR 635-200, 5-13 and 5-17 | January 3, 2019 (expiration: January 3, 2021) | Policy memo to "outline procedures for identification of candidates, mandatory BH screening, evaluation, and administrative review prior to separations of Soldiers under AR 635-200, Chapters 5-13 and 5-17 for BH conditions, not for reasons of other physical health conditions." |
| Army Directive 2018-11 Update to Redesign of Personnel Readiness and Medical Deployability | September 10, 2018 | Directive that "establishes total Army nondeployable goals, makes the Medical Readiness Class (MRC) 4 population deployable, and revises two of the MRCs established in reference 1b to increase the accuracy and consistency of medical readiness reporting for the deployable force." |
| Army Regulation 600-8-101 Personnel—General Personnel Readiness Processing | March 6, 2018 | "This regulation prescribes policy, standards, and requirements for performing the functions of in-processing, out-processing, the Soldier Readiness Program and mobilization processing, and deployment processing." |

**Table A.1—Continued**

| Document Title | Publication Date or Effective Date | Description |
|---|---|---|
| DoD Retention Policy for Non-Deployable Service Members | February 14, 2018 | Policy to "identify changes to military personnel policies necessary to provide more ready and lethal forces." |
| OTSG/MEDCOM Policy Memo 17-079 Behavioral Health eProfiling Standardization Policy | December 28, 2017 (expiration: December 28, 2019) | Policy memo to "provide guidance on issuing profiles for Army personnel with behavioral health (BH) conditions associated treatments to appropriately inform Commanders of duty limitation and treatment support recommendations." |
| Army Regulation 40-501 Medical Services, Standards of Medical Fitness | June 14, 2017 | Regulation that "provides information on medical fitness standards for induction, enlistment, appointment, retention, and related policies and procedures." |
| OTSG/MEDCOM Policy Memo 16-096 Behavioral Health At-Risk Management Policy | November 15, 2016 (expiration: November 15, 2018) | Policy memo that "provides guidance regarding incremental clinical and case management, surveillance, and command communication of behavioral health (BH) cases seen within the Behavioral Health Service Line (BHSL) based on provider risk assessment and available medical and command resources." |
| OTSG/MEDCOM Policy Memo 16-099 Transferring Behavioral Health and Substance Use Disorder Clinical Care or Transitioning Soldiers | November 15, 2016 (expiration: November 15, 2018) | Policy memo to "ensure continuity of care for Soldiers involved in behavioral health (BH) treatment to include Substance Use Disorder Clinical Care (SUDCC) during periods of transition." |
| OTSG/MEDCOM Policy Memo 16-087 Release of Protected Health Information (PHI) to Unit Command Officials | October 18, 2016 (expiration: October 18, 2018) | Policy memo that "presents Office of the Surgeon General and US Army Medical Command (MEDCOM) policy and general guidelines for disclosing and accounting for the minimum necessary Armed Forces members' PHI to be disclosed to commanders and other authorized unit officials." |
| Army Regulation 600-63 Personnel—General Army Health Promotion | April 14, 2015 | This regulation "prescribes policy and sets forth responsibilities for all aspects of the Army Health Promotion Program and implementation of 32 CFR 85." |
| DoD Clinical Practice Guidance for Deployment-Limiting Mental Disorder and Psychotropic Medications | October 7, 2013 | "This memorandum provides clinical practice guidance on limitations of deployment for Service members and DoD civilians who have been diagnosed with mental disorders or who are prescribed psychotropic medication." |

**Table A.1—Continued**

| Document Title | Publication Date or Effective Date | Description |
|---|---|---|
| DoD Instruction 6490.04 Mental Health Evaluations of Members of the Military Services | March 4, 2013 | Instruction "establishing policy, assigning responsibilities, and prescribing procedures for the referral, evaluation, treatment, and medical and command management of Service members who may require assessment for mental health issues, psychiatric hospitalization, and risk of imminent or potential danger to self or others." |
| DoD Instruction 6490.10 Continuity of Behavioral Health Care for Transferring and Transitioning Service Members | March 26, 2012 | Instruction that "establishes policy for the Military Departments, assigns responsibilities, and prescribes guidelines for establishment of Military Department policy and procedures to ensure continuity of behavioral health (BH) care at the losing and gaining installations when Service members transition from one health care provider (HCP) to another when transferring to a new duty station or transitioning out of the Service." |
| DoD Instruction 6490.08 Command Notification Requirements to Dispel Stigma in Providing Mental Health Care to Service Members | August 17, 2011 | Instruction that "establishes policy, assigns responsibilities, and prescribes procedures for health care providers for determining command notification requirements" and to "foster a culture of support in the provision of mental health care and voluntarily sought substance abuse education." |
| DoD Instruction 6490.07 Deployment-Limiting Medical Conditions for Service Members and DoD Civilian Employees | February 5, 2010 | Instruction that "establishes policy, assigns responsibilities, and outlines procedures for ensuring that service members and civilian employees," including those in the U.S. Coast Guard, "are medically able to accomplish their duties in deployed environments." |
| Army Regulation 614-30 Assignments, Details, and Transfers Overseas Service | April 11, 2007 | This regulation "prescribes policies pertinent to overseas permanent change of station moves, overseas tour lengths, overseas tour curtailments, time-on-station, eligibility for overseas service criteria, voluntary and involuntary overseas tour extension, the Overseas Tour Extension Incentive Program, and consecutive overseas tours. It does not prescribe policies pertinent to Soldiers' compensation and entitlements for movement overseas on permanent change of station / temporary change of station." |

**Table A.1—Continued**

| Document Title | Publication Date or Effective Date | Description |
|---|---|---|
| **Combatant Commands Areas of Responsibility-Specific Force Health Protection Guidance** | | |
| U.S. Pacific Command U.S. Forces Korea Reg 40-9 | February 8, 2018 | Lists minimum requirements for personnel who deploy to the U.S. Pacific Command area of responsibility in support of U.S. military operations. |
| U.S. Africa Command, ACI 4200.09 | January 27, 2017 | Lists minimum requirements for personnel who deploy to the U.S. Africa Command area of responsibility in support of U.S. military operations. |
| U.S. Southern Command, SC Reg 40-501 | April 15, 2013 | Lists minimum requirements for personnel who deploy to the U.S. Southern Command area of responsibility in support of U.S. military operations. |
| North American Aerospace Defense Command and U.S. Northern Command, Instruction 44-163 | April 19, 2012 | Lists minimum requirements for personnel who deploy to the North American Aerospace Defense Command / U.S. Northern Command area of responsibility in support of U.S. military operations. |
| U.S. European Command General Administration for Deployment Health Protection Guidance | No date listed | Lists minimum requirements for personnel who deploy to the U.S. European Command area of responsibility in support of U.S. military operations. |
| U.S. Central Command (MOD Thirteen) | No date listed | Lists minimum requirements for personnel who deploy to the U.S. Central Command area of responsibility in support of U.S. military operations. |
| U.S. Central Command (MOD Thirteen) PPG-TAB A | No date listed | "This PPG-TAB A accompanies MOD THIRTEEN, Section 15.C. and provides amplification of the minimal standards of fitness for deployment to the CENTCOM area of responsibility (AOR)." |

# Interview Protocols

### *Army Behavioral Health Expert Interview Guide*

### Interviewee Characteristics

*Structured Questions*

Military service branch:
  **a.** Army
  **b.** Other branch -> not eligible for participation

Status:
  **a.** Active duty
  **b.** DoD or Army civilian
  **c.** Contractor

Rank: _____

What types of role(s) do they have? (mark all that apply)
  **a.** Clinical
  **b.** Administrative
  **c.** Other _____

Do you currently provide behavioral health care at an Army MTF?
  **a.** Yes
  **b.** No

Which types of clinics do you work in? (*circle all that apply*)
  **a.** Primary care
  **b.** Multidisciplinary outpatient BH
  **c.** CAFBHS
  **d.** SUDCC/Army Substance Abuse Program
  **e.** Embedded BH clinic

    **f.** Inpatient/residential
    **g.** Intensive Outpatient Program
    **h.** Other: _____

What type of provider? (*INTERVIEWER: circle the one that aligns most closely*):
    **a.** Psychiatrist
    **b.** Psychologist
    **c.** Licensed social worker
    **d.** Other MA-level counselor
    **e.** Substance use disorder clinical care counselor
    **f.** Psychiatric advanced practice nurse (e.g., psychiatric nurse practitioner)
    **g.** Primary care practitioner
    **h.** Other: _____

Can you tell me about your role?

### Indicators of Readiness for Soldiers in Need of Behavioral Health Care

Prompt: One focus of this project is to identify metrics to assess readiness for soldiers who receive behavioral health care. For this purpose, we have defined *soldier readiness* as the ability to perform mission-essential tasks and deploy without limitations from a behavioral health condition.

    *Probe: Any concerns about this definition?*

Prompt: We are also working to identify metrics to assess family readiness for adult family members who receive behavioral health care. For this purpose, we have defined *family readiness* as the state of being prepared to effectively navigate the challenges of daily living experienced in the unique context of military service, to include: mobility and financial readiness, mobilization and deployment readiness, and personal and family life readiness.

    *Probe: Any concerns about this definition?*

Prompt: Let's focus first on soldiers who receive behavioral health care. What indicators do you believe suggest that Soldiers are *not ready*?

    *Probe: Functional/job-related indicators that would signal that a soldier is not ready/ deployable?*
    *Probe: Interpersonal/interactions with command or other soldiers?*
    *Probe: Related to their behavioral health care (e.g., requirements of treatment, side effects of treatment)?*
    *Probe: Family/relationships? Others?*

Prompt: Now, consider adult family members who receive behavioral health care. What indicators do you believe suggest family member are *not ready*?

>*Probe: Functional/job-related indicators?*
>*Probe: Interpersonal/interactions?*
>*Probe: Family/relationships? Others?*

### Metrics of Readiness Following Behavioral Health Care

Prompt: What existing data could support development of a metric to assess Soldier readiness or family readiness for those who have received behavioral health care? The goal of this metric would be to support evaluating the effectiveness of behavioral health care.

>*Probe: Document each data source (how data are collected, where they reside, what they measure, how frequently are data collected, how closely they assess readiness, who uses/accesses the data). Assess strengths, weaknesses. Show summary list of data sources developed by RAND to address whether additional sources should be included.*

Prompt: Are you aware of any historical use of data to assess readiness of soldiers or families who have received behavioral health care?

>*Probe: Document each data source (how data are collected, where they reside, what they measure, how frequently are data collected, how closely they assess readiness, who uses/accesses the data). Assess strengths, weaknesses.*

### Improving Readiness Assessment

Prompt: What improvements could be made to how readiness is assessed for soldiers who receive behavioral health care?

>*Possible probes: Based on different factors or measures; assessed differently (e.g., more/less frequently); more informed by commanders, behavioral health providers, others.*
>*Possible probes: What new data collection is needed to better assess Soldier and family readiness? What specific measures are needed?*

### Readiness-Related Policies

Prompt: We are collecting readiness-related policies. Are there current or historical policies that we should include in our review?

>*Probe: Include both soldier and family policies.*
>*Probe: May we have a copy of the policies, or can you tell us where we can find them?*

## *Army Behavioral Health Provider Interview Guide*

### *Structured Questions*

Military service branch:
  **a.** Army
  **b.** Other branch -> not eligible for participation

Status:
  **a.** Active duty
  **b.** DoD or Army civilian
  **c.** Contractor

Rank: _____

Do you have clinical role, administrative role, or both?
  **a.** Clinical
  **b.** Administrative
  **c.** Both

Do you currently provide behavioral health care at an Army MTF?
  **a.** Yes
  **b.** No

Which types of clinics do you work in? (*circle all that apply*)
  **a.** Primary care
  **b.** Multidisciplinary outpatient BH
  **c.** CAFBHS
  **d.** SUDCC/Army Substance Abuse Program
  **e.** Embedded BH clinic
  **f.** Inpatient/residential
  **g.** Intensive Outpatient Program
  **h.** Other: _____

What type of provider? (*INTERVIEWER: circle the one that aligns most closely*):
  **a.** Psychiatrist
  **b.** Psychologist
  **c.** Licensed social worker
  **d.** Other MA-level counselor
  **e.** Substance use disorder clinical care counselor
  **f.** Psychiatric advanced practice nurse (e.g., psychiatric nurse practitioner)
  **g.** Primary care practitioner
  **h.** Other: _____

Prompt: Can you tell me your current role/position?

> *Probe: How long you've served in this role?*
> *Probe: What clinical activities are you currently routinely involved in (e.g., intake assessments, psychotherapy, medication management)?*
> *Probe: Do you assess and treat soldiers, family members?*
> *Probe: Do you decide when soldiers are medically ready during or following BH care?*

### Indicators of Readiness for Soldiers in Need of Behavioral Health Care

Prompt: One focus of this project is to identify metrics to assess readiness for soldiers who receive behavioral health care. For this purpose, we have defined *soldier readiness* as the ability to perform mission-essential tasks and deploy without limitations from a behavioral health condition.

> *Probe: Any concerns about this definition?*

Prompt: We are also working to identify metrics to assess family readiness for adult family members who receive behavioral health care. For this purpose, we have defined *family readiness* as the state of being prepared to effectively navigate the challenges of daily living experienced in the unique context of military service, to include: mobility and financial readiness, mobilization and deployment readiness, and personal and family life readiness.

> *Probe: Any concerns about this definition?*

Prompt: Let's focus first on soldiers for whom you provide behavioral health care. What indicators do you observe that suggest that Soldiers are *not ready*?

> *Probe: Functional/job-related indicators that would signal that a soldier is not ready/ deployable?*
> *Probe: Interpersonal/interactions with command or other soldiers?*
> *Probe: Related to their behavioral health care (e.g., requirements of treatment, side effects of treatment)?*
> *Probe: Family/relationships? Others?*

Prompt: Now, consider adult family members who receive behavioral health care. What indicators do you observe that suggest family member are *not ready*?

> *Probe: Functional/job-related indicators?*
> *Probe: Interpersonal/interactions?*
> *Probe: Family/relationships? Others?*

## Assessing Readiness

Prompt: [If the provider indicates above that they make the decision about whether a soldier is ready] What information do you use to assess readiness for soldiers who have received behavioral health care?

> Probe: *Patient-reported measures? Subjective assessment of readiness? Consultation with commander? Collateral information from family or fellow soldiers?*

[If time] Prompt: What influences whether you put a soldier on a profile? Does this vary based on the level or type of profile (temporary vs. permanent)?

> Probe: *Influence of commander? Behavioral health provider?*
> Probe: *Time, competing demands?*
> Probe: *Severity of symptoms? Impact on performing duties?*
> Probe: *Soldier's response to treatment?*

## Soldier Readiness and Interface with Commanders

Prompt: When conducting an assessment or seeing a soldier for behavioral health treatment, do you assess the specific duties that a soldier needs to perform?

> Probe: *Do you communicate with commanders about what an individual soldier needs to be able to do to be considered ready following behavioral health care?*

Prompt: Do you find that your view of readiness is different from that of commanders?

> Probe: *How often have you encountered a situation where you assessed a soldier as ready, but in fact later learned they were not ready (e.g., couldn't perform day-to-day duties, sent home from deployment)? How often have you assessed a soldier as not ready, but the commander overruled you?*
> Probe: *What accounted for the differences in perspective?*
> Probe: *Have you ever felt pressure from a commander to change your assessment?*

## Improving Readiness Assessment

Prompt: In your role as a behavioral health care provider, what improvements could be made to how readiness is assessed for soldiers who receive behavioral health care?

> Possible probes: *based on different factors or specific measures; assessed differently (e.g., more/less frequently); more informed by commanders, behavioral health providers, others.*

# Existing Data Sources

**Table C.1**
**Existing Data Sources Identified**

| Existing Data Source | Description | Reason for Inclusion/Exclusion |
|---|---|---|
| **Database** | | |
| Behavioral Health Readiness Tool (Curley and Warner, 2017) | Tool that can be used to identify service members with BH limitations (based on multiple data sources) who are not on a BH profile | Excluded: This tool is specifically focused on BH profiles, which are covered by the inclusion of eProfile data. This tool has been used in at least one initiative to identify soldiers who should be on a BH profile due to more than minor limitations but are not. Not a tool of readiness tracking. |
| MEDCHART: | | |
|     Health Readiness Record | Repository for Army National Guard and US Army Reserve soldier medical documentation, including BH | Excluded: Includes reservists only |
| MODS | | |
|     Behavioral Health Data Portal (BHDP) (U.S. Army, 2016a) | Module within MODS designed to track BH symptoms to inform treatment and improve BH care | Included: The WRFIS within BHDP measures occupational and personal/social functional impairment for military personnel. Not applicable to family members |
|     eProfile (Womak Army Medical Center, undated) | Tracks soldiers who have been identified as having a permanent or temporary medical condition that may result in medical nonreadiness for deployment | Included: Because service members are placed on a profile when they are not ready, profiles could be used to construct a metric measuring readiness during and following BH care; not applicable to family members |
| Medical Readiness Assessment Tool (U.S. Army, 2015) | Decision support and screening tool designed to proactively identify soldiers and units at risk for targeted management to promote and maintain soldier readiness | Excluded: Model was approximately 80% accurate in predicting ability to deploy in next six months. Based on various health data elements, both BH and non-BH. Model was not widely used. |

**Table C.1—Continued**

| Existing Data Source | Description | Reason for Inclusion/Exclusion |
|---|---|---|
| Medical Readiness Portal (Army Regulation 40-501—Medical Services, Standards of Medical Fitness, 2017) | Combines commander, senior commander, health care, and administrative portals, as well as deployment health assessments and Separation History and Physical Examination applications | Excluded: Served as a new venue for communication between providers and commanders and consolidates applications into portals for ease of use. Most promising elements of Medical Readiness Portal are considered elsewhere in the evaluation of existing data sources (e.g., e-Profile, physical health assessments, Medical Assessment Tool). |
| MHS Data Repository (MHS, 2019) | Patient encounter and dispensed medication data | Excluded: Administrative data about patient encounters (e.g., diagnoses, procedures, labs). The data alone are not enough to measure readiness and lack (uncoded) provider notes that may refer to soldier readiness; family members included. |
| Personnel administrative files | Master or transaction files (e.g., Total Army Personnel Database) that record individual and service characteristics, including PULHES and profiles | Excluded: Secondary indicators of readiness could be measured (e.g., promotion speed), but direct measures of readiness are unlikely to be derived from personnel files. |
| Veterans Tracking Application (VTA) | Integrated Disability Evaluation System, system of record | Excluded: VTA is the system of record for recording transactions of the Integrated Disability Evaluation System for soldiers whose fitness to serve is under valuation. Not all soldiers receiving behavioral health care are in the Integrated Disability Evaluation System. Although soldiers in VTA are not medically ready, VTA would not enable a valid metric of readiness as defined by this project. Family members not in VTA. |
| **Routinely Administered Assessments/Surveys** | | |
| DHA (Psychological Health Center of Excellence [PHCoE], undated a, undated b) | | Excluded: Deployment health assessments (listed below) are tied to deployments and are therefore not administered often enough to measure readiness during and following BH care. Not applicable to family members. |
| Predeployment Health Assessment (Pre-DHA) (PHCoE, undated e) | Self-assessment done within 120 days of the start of a deployment | |

**Table C.1—Continued**

| Existing Data Source | Description | Reason for Inclusion/Exclusion |
|---|---|---|
| Post-deployment Health Assessment (PDHA) (PHCoE, undated c) | Self-assessment completed in-theater or within 30 days of returning home, designed "to review each deployer's current health, mental health or psychosocial issues commonly associated with deployments, special medications taken during the deployment, possible deployment-related occupational/ environmental exposures, and to discuss deployment-related health concerns" | |
| Postdeployment Health Reassessment (PDHRA) (MHS, undated b; PHCoE, undated d) | Self-assessment 3–6 months following deployment | |
| Mental Health Assessment (MHS, undated a) | Postdeployment health screenings designed to identify mental health concerns | |
| Periodic Health Assessment (U.S. Army Human Resources Command, 2019) | Annual preventive screening tool designed to improve reporting and visibility of soldier Individual Medical Readiness; includes self-reported health status, review of medical records, identification, referral for current health, mental health problems, identification and management of occupational health risks, preventive health needs, and identification and development of a plan to manage health risks | Excluded: Periodic Health Assessment occurs annually, which is not frequent enough to be used to construct a readiness measure during and following BH care. Not applicable to family members |
| PULHES | Designation of functional capacity in physical capacity/stamina (P), upper extremities (U), lower extremities (L), hearing/ear (H), eyes (E), psychiatric (S) | Excluded: Score limited to area and level of functional capacity or impairment. No data about impact on duties. |

# Terms Used for Instrument Search

***Solder Readiness Search:*** Military OR soldier OR soldiers OR Army OR Air Force OR Navy OR Marine AND Readiness AND metric OR metrics OR measure OR measures OR survey OR instrument OR profile OR "screening tool" AND "physical functioning" OR "mental functioning" OR "cognitive functioning" OR "social functioning" OR anxiety OR depression OR PTSD OR "duty limitations" OR "return to duty" OR "lost duty time" OR "military absence" OR "Army commitment" OR retention OR "Medical evaluation board" OR "physical evaluation board" OR "other than honorable discharge" OR "serious discharge" OR "military discharge" OR "medical fitness" OR "fitness for duty" OR deployment OR deployments OR deployment health assessment OR deployability OR resilience OR "soldier readiness program" OR sleep OR attention OR memory OR "emotional functions" OR "perceptual functions" OR "higher level cognitive functions" OR "behavioral health" OR "mental health" OR "substance abuse" OR "substance use" OR "alcohol abuse" OR "alcohol use" OR "psychological health" OR "occupational stress" OR "physical health" OR "quality of life" OR "well-being" OR "well being" OR "wellbeing" OR "emotional well-being" OR "emotional well being" OR "emotional wellbeing" OR "morale" OR "moral injury"

***Family Readiness Search:*** "military family" OR "military spouse" AND Readiness AND metric OR metrics OR measure OR measures OR survey OR instrument or profile OR "screening tool" AND "physical functioning" OR "mental functioning" OR "cognitive functioning" OR "social functioning" OR anxiety OR depression OR PTSD OR "military absence" OR "Army commitment" OR "medical fitness" OR deployment OR deployments OR deployability OR resilience OR "soldier readiness program" OR sleep OR attention OR memory OR "emotional functions" OR "perceptual functions" OR "higher level cognitive functions" OR "behavioral health" OR "mental health" OR "substance abuse" OR "substance use" OR "alcohol abuse" OR "alcohol use" OR "psychological health" OR "occupational stress" OR "physical health" OR "quality of life" OR "well-being" OR "well being" OR "wellbeing" OR "emotional well-being" OR "emotional well being" OR "emotional wellbeing" OR "morale" OR "moral injury" OR "family functioning" OR "daily living" OR financial OR social

# Instruments Identified in the Instrument Search

**Table E.1**
**Summary of Instruments**

| Instrument | Description | Domain | Decision During Initial Screening | Reason Excluded |
|---|---|---|---|---|
| Big Five Inventory (Lee, Sudom, and McCreary, 2011) | Assesses personality factors (agreeableness, conscientiousness, extroversion, neuroticism, and openness) | Psychological/ behavioral | Excluded | Exceeded 30-item limit; shorter BFI-10 exists, but not recommended by the BFI originators |
| Brief Insomnia Questionnaire (Klingaman et al., 2018) | Assesses degree of functional impairment due to sleep problems | Physical/ medical | Excluded | Limited focus (sleep) |
| Communication Danger Signs Scale (Erbes et al., 2017) | Assesses frequency of negative interactions between partners | Psychological/ behavioral | Excluded | Limited focus (couple interaction) |
| Confidence Regarding Promotions (Booth-Kewley, Dell'Acqua, and Thomsen, 2017) | Assesses confidence in receiving promotion | Job/duty related | Excluded | Focused on confidence in being promoted and single item |
| Connor-Davidson Resilience Scale (Cunningham et al., 2014) | Assesses resiliency characteristics or qualities across 17 domains of functioning | Job/duty related; psychological/ behavioral | Included | Final exclusion: proprietary tool |
| Coping Strategies Scale (Skomorovsky and Stevens, 2013) | Assesses several coping strategies, including cognitive responses, socioemotional responses, and religious coping | Psychological/ behavioral | Excluded | Exceeded 30-item limit |
| Deployment Risk and Resilience Inventory: Concerns about Life and Family Disruptions Scale (Polusny et al., 2014) | Assesses the extent to which soldiers were worried or concerned about the impact of the pending deployment on their life and family | Psychological/ behavioral | Excluded | Limited focus (deployment) |

**Table E.1—Continued**

| Instrument | Description | Domain | Decision During Initial Screening | Reason Excluded |
|---|---|---|---|---|
| Deployment Risk and Resilience Inventory: Combat Experiences Scale (Polusny et al., 2014) | Assesses objective events and circumstances regarding stereotypical warzone experiences, such as firing on enemies and witnessing casualties of war | Job/duty related | Excluded | Limited focus (combat experiences) |
| Deployment Risk and Resilience Inventory: Social Support Scale (Erbes et al., 2017) | Assesses amount of assistance and encouragement soldiers perceived from unit leaders, other unit members, and military in general | Psychological/ behavioral | Excluded | Limited focus (social support) |
| Deployment Risk and Resilience Inventory: Training and Deployment Preparation (Erbes et al., 2017) | Assesses the extent to which soldiers felt adequately trained to perform duties on deployment, sufficiently advised of upcoming roles, and informed regarding deployment environment | Job/duty related | Excluded | Limited focus (training/ preparedness) |
| Dyadic Adjustment Scale (Erbes et al., 2017) | Assesses agreement between soldiers and partners on specific values, frequency of their positive interactions, and overall degree of happiness in the relationship | Psychological/ behavioral | Excluded | Limited focus (couple interaction) |
| Epworth Sleepiness Scale (Eliasson et al., 2012) | Assesses symptoms of daytime sleepiness | Physical/ medical | Excluded | Limited focus (sleep) |
| Family Index of Coherence (Vasilas, 2010) | Assesses degree to which families feel committed to the military lifestyle and mission, and how much they feel they can count on the military in times of need | Psychological/ behavioral | Excluded | Limited focus (family coherence) |
| Fatigue Scale (Eliasson et al., 2012) | Assesses degree of fatigue | Physical/ medical | Excluded | Limited focus (fatigue) |
| Global Assessment Tool (Lentino et al., 2013) | Assesses soldier's emotional, social, spiritual, and family fitness | Physical/ medical; psychological/ behavioral | Excluded | Exceeded 30-item limit, not linked to individual soldier or spouse |
| Hardiness scale (adapted from Dispositional Resilience Scale) (Lee, Sudom, and McCreary, 2011) | Assesses hardiness | Psychological/ behavioral | Included | Final exclusion: proprietary tool |

**Table E.1—Continued**

| Instrument | Description | Domain | Decision During Initial Screening | Reason Excluded |
|---|---|---|---|---|
| Lost Work Days (Seelig et al., 2016) | Assesses days unable to work or perform your usual activities because of illness or injury | Job/duty related | Excluded | Limited focus (lost work days) |
| Medical Outcomes Study Social Support Survey (Erbes et al., 2017) | Assess social support | Psychological/ behavioral | Excluded | Limited focus (social support) |
| Mediterranean Diet Questionnaire (Eliasson et al., 2012) | Assesses adherence to a Mediterranean-style diet | Physical/ medical | Excluded | Limited focus (diet) |
| Military Hardiness Scale (adapted from Dolan and Adler's 18-item scale) (Skomorovsky and Stevens, 2013) | Assesses military-specific commitment, military-specific challenge, and military-specific control | Job/duty related; psychological/ behavioral | Excluded | Limited focus (military commitment and satisfaction) |
| Navy Quality of Life Survey (Kehle et al., 2011) | Assesses leisure and recreation, friends and friendship, relationship with relatives, marriage/intimate relationships, relationships with children, standard of living, and overall satisfaction with life experiences | Job/duty related; psychological/ behavioral | Excluded | Exceeded 30-item limit |
| Occupational Self-Efficacy (Booth-Kewley, Dell'Acqua, and Thomsen, 2017) | Assesses corpsman's occupational self-efficacy | Psychological/ behavioral; job/duty related | Excluded | Limited focus (corpsman tasks) |
| Organizational Commitment (Booth-Kewley, Dell'Acqua, and Thomsen, 2017) | Assesses affective organizational commitment | Psychological/ behavioral; job/duty related | Excluded | Limited focus (organizational commitment) |
| Perceived Occupational Stress (Booth-Kewley, Dell'Acqua, and Thomsen, 2017) | Assesses degree of stress experienced at work or while carrying out military duties | Job/duty related | Excluded | Limited focus (job stress) |
| Perceived Stress Scale (Eliasson et al., 2012) | Assesses frequency of certain experiences of stress in the last month and the degree to which situations are appraised as stressful | Job/duty related | Excluded | Limited focus (stress) |

**Table E.1—Continued**

| Instrument | Description | Domain | Decision During Initial Screening | Reason Excluded |
|---|---|---|---|---|
| Pittsburgh Sleep Quality Index (Eliasson et al., 2012) | Assesses sleep quality and disturbances | Physical/ medical | Excluded | Limited focus (sleep) |
| Positive and Negative Affect Schedule (Lee, Sudom, and McCreary, 2011) | Assesses positive and negative affect | Physical/ medical; psychological/ behavioral | Excluded | Limited focus (affect) |
| Positive Bonding Scale (Erbes et al., 2017) | Assesses couple's rating of extent of agreement on items related to their friendship, fun, felt support, and intimacy | Psychological/ behavioral | Excluded | Limited focus (couple interaction) |
| Positive Perceptions of Corpsman Training (Booth-Kewley, Dell'Acqua, and Thomsen, 2017) | Assesses the degree the Navy is providing the necessary training to have a successful career as a Corpsman | Job/duty related | Excluded | Limited focus (training) |
| Post-Deployment Social Support Scale (Cunningham et al., 2014) | Assesses postdeployment emotional support and instrumental assistance provided by family, friends, coworkers, employers, and community | Job/duty related; psychological/ behavioral | Excluded | Limited focus (social support) |
| Pre-deployment family stressors scale (Polusny et al., 2014) | Assesses range of stressful events (e.g., loved one passed away, financial problems, relationship infidelity) | Psychological/ behavioral | Excluded | Limited focus (stressful events) |
| Pre-deployment family survey (Polusny et al., 2014) | Assesses family members concerns related to soldier's upcoming deployment | Psychological/ behavioral | Excluded | Limited focus (parental concerns) |
| Preservice Motivation to Become a Corpsman (Booth-Kewley, Dell'Acqua. and Thomsen, 2017) | Assesses preservice motivation to become a corpsman | Job/duty related | Excluded | Limited focus (vocational interest) |
| Prior Stressors Scale (Erbes et al., 2017) | Assesses traumatic or stressful events | Psychological/ behavioral | Excluded | Limited focus (prior stressful events) |
| Revised Life Orientation Test (Lee, Sudom, and McCreary, 2011) | Assesses optimism | Psychological/ behavioral | Excluded | Limited focus (optimism) |

**Table E.1—Continued**

| Instrument | Description | Domain | Decision During Initial Screening | Reason Excluded |
|---|---|---|---|---|
| Satisfaction with Life Scale (Skomorovsky and Stevens, 2013) | Assesses global life satisfaction | Psychological/ behavioral | Excluded | Limited focus (life satisfaction) |
| Self-esteem measure (Lee, Sudom and McCreary, 2011) | Assesses self-esteem | Psychological/ behavioral | Excluded | Limited focus (self-esteem) |
| Self-Rated General Health (Seelig et al., 2016) | Assesses self-report of general health | Physical/ medical | Excluded | Limited focus (single item of global health) |
| Self-report health status (Saffari et al., 2015) | Assesses perceived health status | Physical/ medical | Excluded | Limited focus (single item of global health) |
| Short form-36 health survey (Saffari et al., 2015) | Assesses eight domains: physical activity, role limitations because of physical difficulties, bodily pain, general health, vitality, social functioning, role limitations because of emotional difficulties, and mental health | Physical/ medical; psychological/ behavioral | Excluded | Exceeded 30-item limit |
| Sleep duration (Seelig et al., 2016) | Assesses average nightly sleep | Physical/ medical | Excluded | Limited focus (sleep) |
| Sleep quality (short version Pittsburgh Insomnia Rating Scale) (Lentino et al., 2013) | Assesses sleep quality | Physical/ medical | Excluded | Limited focus (sleep) |
| Sleep questionnaire (Miller, Shattuck, and Matsangas, 2011) | Assesses sleep hygiene during deployment | Physical/ medical | Excluded | Limited focus (sleep) |
| Social Adjustment Scale-Self-Report (Kehle et al., 2011) | Assesses functioning in six areas: work, social and leisure activities, relationships with family, role as marital partner, parental role, and role within the family unit including economic functioning | Job/duty related; psychological/ behavioral | Excluded | Exceeded 30-item limit |
| Social Readjustment Rating Scale— Schedule of Recent Experiences (Cunningham et al., 2014) | Assesses exposure to life events commonly reported as stressful and that also require personal adjustment | Job/duty related; psychological/ behavioral | Excluded | Exceeded 30-item limit |

**Table E.1—Continued**

| Instrument | Description | Domain | Decision During Initial Screening | Reason Excluded |
|---|---|---|---|---|
| Unit leadership (Klingaman et al., 2018) | Assesses unit member and leadership support | Job/duty related; psychological/ behavioral | Excluded | Limited focus (unit support) |
| Social Support for Corpsman Career (Booth-Kewley, Dell'Acqua, and Thomsen, 2017) | Assesses soldiers support from family and friends for their Navy career plans | Job/duty related | Excluded | Limited focus (career support) |
| Social Support Index (Vasilas, 2010) | Assesses the degree to which families are integrated into the community | Psychological/ behavioral | Excluded | Limited focus (social support) |
| Social Support Survey (Lee, Sudom, and McCreary, 2011) | Assesses various types of social support | Psychological/ behavioral | Excluded | Limited focus (social support) |
| Task-Specific Self-Efficacy (Booth-Kewley, Dell'Acqua, and Thomsen, 2017) | Confidence in one's ability to execute specific occupational tasks | Job/duty related; psychological/ behavioral | Excluded | Limited focus (specific skill competency) |

NOTE: Citation refers to the article of origin from the instrument search and not the instrument reference.

# Instruments from Supplemental Search

**Table F.1**
**Summary of Instruments from Supplemental Search**

| Instrument | Description | Source of Recommendation | Decision During Initial Screening | Reason Excluded |
|---|---|---|---|---|
| Ability to Participate in Social Roles and Activities–Short Form 8a (American Psychological Association, 2019) | Level of trouble with leisure, family, work, and social activities (PROMIS item bank: 8 items) | American Psychological Association | Excluded | Primary focus on social roles |
| Daily Living Activities (Scott and Presmanes, 2001) | Impact of physical and mental health limitations on 20 activities (20 items) | Kennedy Forum | Excluded | Provider assessment, focus on severe mental disorders |
| Functional Health Survey (Institute for Healthcare Improvement, 2019a) | Patient self-report of physical and emotional health (6 items) | Institute for Healthcare Improvement | Excluded | Focus on physical and mental health limitations, no social functioning |
| International Classification of Functioning, Disability, and Health Checklist (World Health Organization, undated) | Functioning, disability, and health; coded with body functioning, body structure, activities and participation, and environmental factors with qualifiers denoting magnitude | World Health Organization | Excluded | Provider assessment, complex coding, exceeded 30 items |
| PROMIS (Northwestern University, 2019) | | | | |
| PROMIS Global Health | Patient self-report of general health, physical health, mental health, social/work, fatigue, pain (10 items) | | | |
| PROMIS-29 Profile | A collection of 4-item short forms assessing physical functioning, anxiety, depression, fatigue, pain, sleep disturbance, social roles (29 items) | Subject-matter expert recommendation | Included | Final exclusion: Focus on difficulties due to physical/mental health conditions |

**Table F.1—Continued**

| Instrument | Description | Source of Recommendation | Decision During Initial Screening | Reason Excluded |
|---|---|---|---|---|
| Short Form Survey, Medical Outcomes Study (including related Veteran RAND surveys) (Ware, Sherbourne, and Davies, 1992) | Patient self-report of physical and mental health, pain, occupational, social (20 items) | Subject-matter expert recommendation | Excluded | Complicated scoring |
| Social Support Survey, Medical Outcomes Outcome Study (Moser et al., 2012) | Patient self-report measure of social support (8 or 19 items) | International Consortium for Health Outcomes Measurement | Excluded | Limited to social support |
| World Health Organization Disability Assessment Schedule, 2.0 (World Health Organization, 2010) | Patient self-report of physical, emotional, social/occupational functioning (12 items) | International Consortium for Health Outcomes Measurement and Kennedy Forum | Included | Final exclusion: Focus on difficulties due to physical/mental health conditions |

# References

Adirim, Terry, "A Military Health System for the Twenty-First Century," *Health Affairs*, Vol. 38, No. 8, 2019, pp. 1268–1273.

Adrian, Amanda L., Amy B. Adler, Jeffrey L. Thomas, and Thomas W. Britt, "Integrating New Soldiers: The Role of Leaders and Unit Members," *Military Psychology*, Vol. 30, No. 2, 2018, pp. 131–141.

American Psychological Association, "Mental and Behavioral Health Registry (MBHR)," webpage, 2019. As of August 20, 2019:
https://www.apaservices.org/practice/reimbursement/health-registry/measures

Army Regulation 40-501, *Medical Services, Standards of Medical Fitness*, Washington, D.C.: Headquarters, Department of the Army, 2017.

Bartone, Paul T., "Test-Retest Reliability of the Dispositional Resilience Scale-15: A Brief Hardiness Scale," *Psychological Reports*, Vol. 101, No. 3, 2007, pp. 943–944.

———, "Hardiness-Resilience: Research and Background Information on the Dispositional Resilience Scale (DRS)," webpage, September 20, 2008. As of August 6, 2019:
https://www.hardiness-resilience.com

Booth-Kewley, Stephanie, Renée G. Dell'Acqua, and Cynthia J. Thomsen, "Factors Affecting Organizational Commitment in Navy Corpsmen," *Military Medicine*, Vol. 182, No. 7, 2017, pp. e1794–e1800.

Bradshaw, Carmel, Sandra Atkinson, and Owen Doody, "Employing a Qualitative Description Approach in Health Care Research," *Global Qualitative Nursing Research*, Vol. 4, 2017, pp. 1–8. As of March 14, 2020:
https://doi.org/10.1177/2333393617742282

CDRISC, homepage, undated. As of August 6, 2019:
http://www.cd-risc.com

Cella, David, William Riley, Arthur Stone, Nan Rothrock, Bryce Reeve, Susan Yount, Dagmar Amtmann, Rita Bode, Daniel Buysse, and Seung Choi, "Initial Adult Health Item Banks and First Wave Testing of the Patient-Reported Outcomes Measurement Information System (PROMIS™) Network: 2005–2008," *Journal of Clinical Epidemiology*, Vol. 63, No. 11, 2010, pp. 1179–1194.

Center for Clinical Standards and Quality, Centers for Medicare and Medicaid Services, *CMS Quality Measure Development Plan 2019 Annual Report*, Baltimore, Md.: Centers for Medicare and Medicaid Services, 2019. As of March 14, 2020:
https://www.cms.gov/Medicare/Quality-Payment-Program/Measure-Development/Measure-development

Chairman of the Joint Chiefs of Staff Instruction 3405.01, *Chairman's Total Force Fitness Framework*, September 1, 2011. As of August 2, 2019:
https://www.jcs.mil/Portals/36/Documents/Library/Instructions/3405_01.pdf?ver=2016-02-05-175032-517

Chandra, Anita, Sandraluz Lara-Cinisomo, Lisa H. Jaycox, Terri Tanielian, Rachel M. Burns, Teague Ruder, and Bing Han, "Children on the Homefront: The Experience of Children from Military Families," *Pediatrics*, Vol. 125, No. 1, 2010, pp. 16–25.

Connor, Kathryn M., and Jonathan R. T. Davidson, "Development of a New Resilience Scale: The Connor-Davidson Resilience Scale (CD-RISC)," *Depression and Anxiety*, Vol. 18, No. 2, 2003, pp. 76–82.

Cronrath, Corey M., Joseph Venezia, Titus J. Rund, Timothy H. Cho, Nicole M. Solana, and Jennifer A. Benincasa, "Medical Redeployment in Soldiers With and Without Medical Deployment Waivers," *Military Medicine*, Vol. 182, No. 3–4, 2017, pp. e1704–e1708.

Crouch, Coleen, Justin M. Curley, Jamie T. Carreno, and Joshua E. Wilk, "Return to Duty Practices of Army Behavioral Health Providers in Garrison," *Military Medicine*, Vol. 183, No. 11–12, 2018, pp. e617–e623.

Cunningham, Craig A., Bryan A. Weber, Beverly L. Roberts, Tracy S. Hejmanowski, Wayne D. Griffin, and Barbara J. Lutz, "The Role of Resilience and Social Support in Predicting Postdeployment Adjustment in Otherwise Healthy Navy Personnel," *Military Medicine*, Vol. 179, No. 9, 2014, pp. 979–985.

Curley, Justin M., *The Behavioral Health Readiness Evaluation and Decision-Making Instrument (B-REDI) Study*, Kissimmee, Fla.: Military Health System Research Symposium, August 2019.

Curley, Justin M., Coleen Crouch, and Joshua E. Wilk, "Minor Behavioral Health Readiness and Profiling Barriers in the US Army," *Military Medicine*, Vol. 183, No. 9–10, 2018, pp. e297–e301.

Curley, Justin M., and Christopher H. Warner, "Improving Awareness of Behavioral Health Readiness," *Military Medicine*, Vol. 182, No. 7, 2017, pp. e1738–e1746.

Defense Health Agency, "Defense Health Agency Procedural Instruction 6490.01: Behavioral Health (BH) Treatment and Outcomes Monitoring," 2018. As of August 2, 2019:
https://health.mil/Search-Results?query=6490.01

———, "DHA Procedures Manual, Clinical Quality Management in the Military Health System, Number 6025.13, Volumes 6 and 7," 2019. As of September 5, 2019:
https://www.Health.mil/Reference-Center/Policies

Department of Defense, "Report to Armed Services Committees of the Senate and House of Representatives: Section 729 of the National Defense Authorization Act for Fiscal Year 2016 (Public Law 114-92); Plan for Development of Procedures to Measure Data on Mental Health Care Provided by the Department of Defense," September 2016. As of May 18, 2018:
https://health.mil/Reference-Center/Reports/2016/09/13/Plan-for-Development-of-Procedures-to-Measure

Department of Defense Instruction 1342.22, *Military Family Readiness*, Washington, D.C.: U.S. Department of Defense, July 3, 2012. As of August 2, 2019:
https://www.esd.whs.mil/Portals/54/Documents/DD/issuances/dodi/134222p.pdf

Department of Defense Instruction 6025.19, *Individual Medical Readiness (IMR)*, Washington, D.C.: U.S. Department of Defense, June 9, 2014. As of August 5, 2019:
https://www.esd.whs.mil/Portals/54/Documents/DD/issuances/dodi/602519p.pdf

Department of Defense Instruction 6490.07, *Deployment-Limiting Medical Conditions for Service Members and DoD Civilian Employees*, Washington, D.C.: U.S. Department of Defense, February 5, 2010. As of March 15, 2020:
https://www.esd.whs.mil/Portals/54/Documents/DD/issuances/dodi/649007p.pdf

Deployment Health Clinical Center, *Mental Health Disorder Prevalence Among Active Duty Service Members in the Military Health System, Fiscal Years 2005–2016*, Falls Church, Va.: Deployment Health Clinical Center, Psychological Health Center of Excellence, 2017. As of August 2, 2019:
https://www.pdhealth.mil/sites/default/files/images/mental-health-disorder-prevalence-among-active -duty-service-members-508.pdf

DoD—*See* Department of Defense.

Donabedian, Avedis, "The Quality of Care: How Can It Be Assessed?" *JAMA*, Vol. 260, No. 12, 1988, pp. 1743–1748.

Duffy, Farifteh, "Contractor Center for Military Psychiatry and Neuroscience Walter Reed Army Institute of Research," email to Kimberly Hepner, July 18, 2019.

Eaton, Karen M., Charles W. Hoge, Stephen C. Messer, Allison A. Whitt, Oscar A. Cabrera, Dennis McGurk, Anthony Cox, and Carl A. Castro, "Prevalence of Mental Health Problems, Treatment Need, and Barriers to Care Among Primary Care–Seeking Spouses of Military Service Members Involved in Iraq and Afghanistan Deployments," *Military Medicine*, Vol. 173, No. 11, 2008, pp. 1051–1056.

Eliasson, Arn, Mariam Kashani, Georgia Dela Cruz, and Marina Vernalis, "Readiness and Associated Health Behaviors and Symptoms in Recently Deployed Army National Guard Soldiers," *Military Medicine*, Vol. 177, No. 11, 2012, pp. 1254–1260.

Erbes, Christopher R., Mark Kramer, Paul A. Arbisi, David DeGarmo, and Melissa A. Polusny, "Characterizing Spouse/Partner Depression and Alcohol Problems over the Course of Military Deployment," *Journal of Consulting and Clinical Psychology*, Vol. 85, No. 4, 2017, pp. 297–308.

Harding, Kelli Jane, A. John Rush, Melissa Arbuckle, Madhukar H. Trivedi, and Harold Alan Pincus, "Measurement-Based Care in Psychiatric Practice: A Policy Framework for Implementation," *Journal of Clinical Psychiatry*, Vol. 72, No. 8, 2011, pp. 1136–1143.

Hawkins, Stacy Ann, Annie Condon, Jacob N. Hawkins, Kristine Liu, Yxsel Melendrez Ramirez, Marisa M. Nihill, and Jackson Tolins, *What We Know About Military Family Readiness: Evidence from 2007–2017*, Monterey, Calif.: Research Facilitation Laboratory, 2018. As of August 5, 2019:
https://apps.dtic.mil/dtic/tr/fulltext/u2/1050341.pdf

Hays, Ron D., Jakob B. Bjorner, Dennis A. Revicki, Karen L. Spritzer, and David Cella, "Development of Physical and Mental Health Summary Scores from the Patient-Reported Outcomes Measurement Information System (PROMIS) Global Items," *Quality of Life Research*, Vol. 18, No. 7, 2009, pp. 873–880.

Hepner, Kimberly A., Coreen Farris, Carrie M. Farmer, Praise O. Iyiewuare, Terri Tanielian, Asa Wilks, Michael Robbins, Susan M. Paddock, and Harold Alan Pincus, *Delivering Clinical Practice Guideline–Concordant Care for PTSD and Major Depression in Military Treatment Facilities*, Santa Monica, Calif.: RAND Corporation, RR-1692-OSD, 2017. As of September 23, 2019:
https://www.rand.org/pubs/research_reports/RR1692.html

Herrell, Richard K., Edward N. Edens, Lyndon A. Riviere, Jeffrey L. Thomas, Paul D. Bliese, and Charles W. Hoge, "Assessing Functional Impairment in a Working Military Population: The Walter Reed Functional Impairment Scale," *Psychological Services*, Vol. 11, No. 3, 2014, p. 254.

Hoge, Charles W., Christopher G. Ivany, Edward A. Brusher, Millard D. Brown III, John C. Shero, Amy B. Adler, Christopher H. Warner, and David T. Orman, "Transformation of Mental Health Care for US Soldiers and Families During the Iraq and Afghanistan Wars: Where Science and Politics Intersect," *American Journal of Psychiatry*, Vol. 173, No. 4, 2015, pp. 334–343.

Institute for Healthcare Improvement, "Functional Health Survey–6 (FHS-6) Patient Questionnaires," 2019a. As of August 6, 2019:
http://www.ihi.org/resources/Pages/Measures/FHS6PatientQuestionnaires.aspx

———, "Quality Improvement Essentials Toolkit," 2019b. As of August 21, 2019:
http://www.ihi.org/resources/Pages/Tools/Quality-Improvement-Essentials-Toolkit.aspx

The Joint Commission, "Revised Outcome Measures Standard: Behavioral Health Care Accreditation Program," undated. As of August 21, 2019:
https://www.jointcommission.org/assets/1/6/Revised_Outcome_Measures_Standard.pdf

———, homepage, 2020. As of August 5, 2019:
http://www.jointcommision.org/

Kehle, Shannon M., Madhavi K. Reddy, Amanda G. Ferrier-Auerbach, Christopher R. Erbes, Paul A. Arbisi, and Melissa A. Polusny, "Psychiatric Diagnoses, Comorbidity, and Functioning in National Guard Troops Deployed to Iraq," *Journal of Psychiatric Research*, Vol. 45, No. 1, 2011, pp. 126–132.

Klingaman, Elizabeth A., Janeese A. Brownlow, Elaine M. Boland, Caterina Mosti, and Philip R. Gehrman, "Prevalence, Predictors and Correlates of Insomnia in US Army Soldiers," *Journal of Sleep Research*, Vol. 27, No. 3, 2018, p. e12612.

Larson, Mary Jo, Beth A. Mohr, Rachel Sayko Adams, Grant Ritter, Jennifer Perloff, Thomas V. Williams, Diana D. Jeffery, and Christopher Tompkins, "Association of Military Deployment of a Parent or Spouse and Changes in Dependent Use of Health Care Services," *Medical Care*, Vol. 50, No. 9, 2012, pp. 821–828.

Lee, Jennifer E. C., Kerry A. Sudom, and Donald R. McCreary, "Higher-Order Model of Resilience in the Canadian Forces," *Canadian Journal of Behavioural Science / Revue canadienne des sciences du comportement*, Vol. 43, No. 3, 2011, p. 222.

Lee, Yena, Joshua D. Rosenblat, Jung Goo Lee, Nicole E. Carmona, Mehala Subramaniapillai, Margarita Shekotikhina, Rodrigo B. Mansur, Elisa Brietzke, Jae-Hon Lee, Roger C. Ho, Samantha J. Yim, and Roger S. McIntyre, "Efficacy of Antidepressants on Measures of Workplace Functioning in Major Depressive Disorder: A Systematic Review," *Journal of Affective Disorders*, Vol. 227, February, 2018, pp. 406–415.

Lentino, Cynthia V., Dianna L. Purvis, Kaitlin J. Murphy, and Patricia A. Deuster, "Sleep as a Component of the Performance Triad: The Importance of Sleep in a Military Population," *US Army Medical Department Journal*, 2013, pp. 98–108.

Lester, Patricia, Kris Peterson, James Reeves, Larry Knauss, Dorie Glover, Catherine Mogil, Naihua Duan, William Saltzman, Robert Pynoos, and Katherine Wilt, "The Long War and Parental Combat Deployment: Effects on Military Children and At-Home Spouses," *Journal of the American Academy of Child and Adolescent Psychiatry*, Vol. 49, No. 4, 2010, pp. 310–320.

Martinez, Ruben G., Cara C. Lewis, and Bryan J. Weiner, "Instrumentation Issues in Implementation Science," *Implementation Science: IS*, Vol. 9, 2014. As of March 14, 2020:
https://doi.org/10.1186/s13012-014-0118-8

Meadows, Sarah O., Megan K. Beckett, Kirby Bowling, Daniela Golinelli, Michael P. Fisher, Laurie T. Martin, Lisa S. Meredith, and Karen Chan Osilla, "Family Resilience in the Military: Definitions, Models, and Policies," *RAND Health Quarterly*, Vol. 5, No. 3, 2016.

Meadows, Sarah O., Charles C. Engel, Rebecca L. Collins, Robin L. Beckman, Matthew Cefalu, Jennifer Hawes-Dawson, Molly Doyle, Amii M. Kress, Lisa Sontag-Padilla, Rajeev Ramchand, and Kayla M. Williams, "2015 Department of Defense Health Related Behaviors Survey (HRBS)," *RAND Health Quarterly*, Vol. 8, No. 2, 2018, p. 5.

MHS—*See* Military Health System.

Military Health System, "Mental Health Assessment," webpage, undated a. As of August 6, 2019: https://health.mil/Military-Health-Topics/Health-Readiness/Reserve-Health-Readiness-Program/Our-Services/Mental-Health-Assessment

———, "Post-Deployment Health Reassessment," webpage, undated b. As of August 6, 2019: https://health.mil/Military-Health-Topics/Health-Readiness/Reserve-Health-Readiness-Program/Our-Services/PDHRA

———, "Military Health System Data Repository," webpage, 2019. As of August 21, 2019: https://www.health.mil/Military-Health-Topics/Technology/Clinical-Support/Military-Health-System-Data-Repository

Miller, Nita Lewis, Lawrence G. Shattuck, and Panagiotis Matsangas, "Sleep and Fatigue Issues in Continuous Operations: A Survey of US Army Officers," *Behavioral Sleep Medicine*, Vol. 9, No. 1, 2011, pp. 53–65.

Milley, Mark A., General, U.S. Army, "Army Readiness Guidance, Calendar Year 2016–17," memorandum to all Army leaders, 2016. As of August 21, 2019: https://www.army.mil/e2/downloads/rv7/standto/docs/army_readiness_guidance.pdf

Moser, André, Andreas E. Stuck, Rebecca A. Silliman, Patricia A. Ganz, and Kerri M. Clough-Gorr, "The Eight-Item Modified Medical Outcomes Study Social Support Survey: Psychometric Evaluation Showed Excellent Performance," *Journal of Clinical Epidemiology*, Vol. 65, No. 10, 2012, pp. 1107–1116.

National Academies of Sciences, Engineering, and Medicine, *Strengthening the Military Family Readiness System for a Changing American Society*, Washington, D.C.: National Academies Press, 2019. As of August 5, 2019: https://www.nap.edu/catalog/25380/strengthening-the-military-family-readiness-system-for-a-changing-american-society

National Health Service, East London Foundation Trust, "The Model for Understanding Success in Quality (MUSIQ)," webpage, 2019. As of August 21, 2019: https://qi.elft.nhs.uk/resource/the-model-for-understanding-success-in-quality-2/

National Quality Forum, *The ABCs of Measurement*, Washington, D.C.: National Quality Forum, 2018. As of August 5, 2019: http://www.qualityforum.org/Measuring_Performance/ABCs_of_Measurement.aspx

———, "NQF Measure #1884," webpage, 2019a. As of August 29, 2019: https://www.qualityforum.org/QPS/QPSTool.aspx

———, "Quality Positioning System," webpage, 2019b. As of August 29, 2019: https://www.qualityforum.org/QPS/QPSTool.aspx

Neergaard, Mette Asbjoern, Frede Olesen, Rikke Sand Andersen, and Jens Sondergaard, "Qualitative Description—the Poor Cousin of Health Research?" *BMC Medical Research Methodology*, Vol. 9, No. 1, 2009, p. 52.

Nindl, Bradley C., Daniel C. Billing, Jace R. Drain, Meaghan E. Beckner, Julie Greeves, Herbert Groeller, Hilde K. Teien, Samuele Marcora, Anthony Moffitt, and Tara Reilly, "Perspectives on Resilience for Military Readiness and Preparedness: Report of an International Military Physiology Roundtable," *Journal of Science and Medicine in Sport*, Vol. 21, No. 11, 2018, pp. 1116–1124.

Northwestern University, "Health Measures—PROMIS," webpage, 2019. As of August 6, 2019:
http://www.healthmeasures.net/explore-measurement-systems/promis

PHCoE—*See* Psychological Health Center of Excellence.

Polusny, Melissa A., Christopher R. Erbes, Emily Hagel Campbell, Hannah Fairman, Mark Kramer, and Alexandria K. Johnson, "Pre-Deployment Well-Being Among Single and Partnered National Guard Soldiers: The Role of Their Parents, Social Support, and Stressors," in Shelley MacDermid Wadsworth and David S. Riggs, eds., *Military Deployment and Its Consequences for Families*, New York: Springer, 2014, pp. 151–172.

Psychological Health Center of Excellence, "Deployment Health Assessments," webpage, undated a. As of August 6, 2019:
https://www.pdhealth.mil/clinical-guidance/deployment-health-assessments

———, "Periodic Health Assessment," webpage, undated b. As of August 21, 2019:
https://www.health.mil/Military-Health-Topics/Health-Readiness/
Reserve-Health-Readiness-Program/Our-Services/PHA

———, "Post-Deployment Health Assessment," webpage, undated c. As of August 6, 2019:
https://health.mil/Military-Health-Topics/Combat-Support/Public-Health/Deployment-Health

———, "Post-Deployment Health Reassessment," webpage, undated d. As of August 6, 2019:
https://health.mil/Military-Health-Topics/Health-Readiness/Reserve-Health-Readiness-Program/
Our-Services/PDHRA

———, "Pre-Deployment Health Assessment," webpage, undated e. As of August 6, 2019:
https://health.mil/Military-Health-Topics/Combat-Support/Public-Health/Deployment-Health

Saffari, Mohsen, Harold G. Koenig, Amir H. Pakpour, and Mohammad Gamal Sehlo, "Health Related Quality of Life Among Military Personnel: What Socio-Demographic Factors Are Important?" *Applied Research in Quality of Life*, Vol. 10, No. 1, 2015, pp. 63–76.

Scott, Roger L., and Willa S. Presmanes, "Reliability and Validity of the Daily Living Activities Scale: A Functional Assessment Measure for Severe Mental Disorders," *Research on Social Work Practice*, Vol. 11, No. 3, 2001, pp. 373–389.

Secretary of the Army, "Army Directive 2018-11 Update to Redesign of Personnel Readiness and Medical Deployability," 2018. As of August 5, 2019:
https://armypubs.army.mil/epubs/DR_pubs/DR_a/pdf/web/ARN12904_AD2018_11_Final.pdf

Seelig, Amber D., Isabel G. Jacobson, Carrie J. Donoho, Daniel W. Trone, Nancy F. Crum-Cianflone, and Thomas J. Balkin, "Sleep and Health Resilience Metrics in a Large Military Cohort," *Sleep*, Vol. 39, No. 5, 2016, pp. 1111–1120.

Skomorovsky, Alla, and Sonya Stevens, "Testing a Resilience Model Among Canadian Forces Recruits," *Military Medicine*, Vol. 178, No. 8, 2013, pp. 829–837.

Slade, Mike, Paul McCrone, Elizabeth Kuipers, Morven Leese, Sharon Cahill, Alberto Parabiaghi, Stefan Priebe, and Graham Thornicroft, "Use of Standardised Outcome Measures in Adult Mental Health Services: Randomised Controlled Trial," *British Journal of Psychiatry*, Vol. 189, No. 4, 2006, pp. 330–336.

Spiro, A., III, W. H. Rogers, S. Qian, and L. Kazis, *Imputing Physical and Mental Summary Scores (PCS and MCS) for the "Veterans RAND 12 Item Health Survey" (VR-12—Formerly Called the Veterans SF-12) in the Context of Missing Data*, Baltimore, Md.: Center for Medicare and Medicaid Services, National Committee for Quality Assurance, 2004.

Spitzer, Robert L., Kurt Kroenke, Janet B. W. Williams, and Patient Health Questionnaire Primary Care Study Group, "Validation and Utility of a Self-Report Version of PRIME-MD: The PHQ Primary Care Study," *JAMA*, Vol. 282, No. 18, 1999, pp. 1737–1744.

Steenkamp, Maria M., Nida H. Corry, Meng Qian, Meng Li, Hope Seib McMaster, John A. Fairbank, Valerie A. Stander, Laura Hollahan, and Charles R. Marmar, "Prevalence of Psychiatric Morbidity in United States Military Spouses: The Millennium Cohort Family Study," *Depression and Anxiety*, Vol. 35, No. 9, 2018, pp. 815–829.

Stein, Bradley D., Alyce S. Adams, and David A. Chambers, "A Learning Behavioral Health Care System: Opportunities to Enhance Research," *Psychiatric Services*, Vol. 67, No. 9, 2016, pp. 1019–1022.

Trivedi, Madhukar H., David W. Morris, Stephen R. Wisniewski, Ira Lesser, Andrew A. Nierenberg, Ella Daly, Benji T. Kurian, Bradley N. Gaynes, G. K. Balasubramani, and A. John Rush, "Increase in Work Productivity of Depressed Individuals with Improvement in Depressive Symptom Severity," *American Journal of Psychiatry*, Vol. 170, No. 6, 2013, pp. 633–641.

U.S. Army, "Medical Readiness Assessment Tool (MRAT)," webpage, 2015. As of August 21, 2019: https://www.army.mil/article/159086/medical_readiness_assessment_tool_mrat

———, "Behavioral Data Health Portal," webpage, 2016a. As of August 5, 2019: https://armymedicine.health.mil/Behavioral-Health/Behavioral-Data-Health-Portal

———, *US Army Memorandum: Behavioral Health At-Risk Management Policy, Policy Memo 16-096*, 2016b.

———, *US Army Memorandum: Behavioral Health eProfiling Standardization Policy, Policy Memo 17-079*, 2017.

U.S. Army Human Resources Command, "Periodic Health Assessment," webpage, 2019. As of August 21, 2019: https://www.hrc.army.mil/content/Periodic%20Health%20Assessment%20(PHA)

U.S. Army Public Health Center, *2018 Health of the Force*, Gunpowder, Md.: Army Public Health Center, 2018. As of August 2, 2019: https://phc.amedd.army.mil/Periodical%20Library/2018HealthoftheForceReport.pdf

U.S. Central Command, "231245Z MAR 17 MOD Thirteen to USCENTCOM Individual Protection and Individual-Unit Deployment Policy," 2017.

Vasilas, Cynthia Nikki, *Critical Needs and Level of Support for the Military Spouse: A Comparative Study of the National Guard and Active Army During the Iraq war (Dissertation)*, Auburn, Ala.: Auburn University, 2010.

Ware, John E., Cathy D. Sherbourne, and Allyson R. Davies, "Developing and Testing the MOS 20-Item Short-Form Health Survey: A General Population Application," in Anita L. Stewart and John E. Ware, eds., *Measuring Functioning and Well-Being: The Medical Outcomes Study Approach*, Durham, N.C.: Duke University Press, 1992, pp. 277–290.

Watkins, Daphne C., "Rapid and Rigorous Qualitative Data Analysis: The 'RADaR' Technique for Applied Research," *International Journal of Qualitative Methods*, Vol. 16, No. 1, 2017. As of March 14, 2020: https://doi.org/10.1177%2F1609406917712131

Wooten, Nikki R., Jordan A. Brittingham, Ronald O. Pitner, Abbas S. Tavakoli, Diana D. Jeffery, and K. Sue Haddock, "Purchased Behavioral Health Care Received by Military Health System Beneficiaries in Civilian Medical Facilities, 2000–2014," *Military Medicine*, Vol. 183, No. 7–8, 2018, pp. e278–e290.

Womak Army Medical Center, homepage, undated. As of August 5, 2019:
https://www.wamc.amedd.army.mil/HealthcareServices/SitePages/e-Profile.aspx

World Health Organization, "ICF Checklist, Version 2.1a, Clinician Form for International Classification of Functioning, Disability and Health," undated. As of August 6, 2019:
https://www.who.int/classifications/icf/icfchecklist.pdf?ua=1

———, *Measuring Health and Disability: Manual for WHO Disability Assessment Schedule WHODAS 2.0*, Geneva, Switzerland: World Health Organization, 2010.

Wright, Caroline V., Carol Goodheart, David Bard, Bruce L. Bobbitt, Zeeshan Butt, Kathleen Lysell, Dean McKay, and Kari Stephens, "Promoting Measurement-Based Care and Quality Measure Development: The APA Mental and Behavioral Health Registry Initiative," *Psychological Services*, 2019, advance online publication. As of March 14, 2020:
https://psycnet.apa.org/doi/10.1037/ser0000347